A Workbook of Manual Therapy Techniques
for the Vertebral Column
and Pelvic Girdle

A Workbook of Manual Therapy Techniques for the Vertebral Column and Pelvic Girdle

2nd Edition
Fully Revised

Diane G. Lee BSR MCPA COMP
Instructor, Orthopaedic Division C.P.A.
Examiner, Canadian Orthopaedic Manipulative Physiotherapists

Mari C. Walsh MCPA MISCP COMP
Instructor, Orthopaedic Division C.P.A.
Examiner, Canadian Orthopaedic Manipulative Physiotherapists

Canadian Cataloguing in Publication Data

Lee, Diane.
  A workbook of manual therapy techniques for the vertebral
column and pelvic girdle

  ISBN 1-55056-429-3

  1. Spinal adjustment – Handbooks, manuals, etc. 2.
Manipulation (Therapeutics) – Handbooks, manuals, etc. I.
Walsh, Mari C., 1951- II. Title.
RZ242.9.L43 1996   615.8'2   C96-910175-9

Printed in Canada by

Friesen Printers, Altona, Manitoba

PREFACE TO THE FIRST EDITION

Musculoskeletal disorders can be effectively treated with physiotherapy, including mobilization (active and passive), stabilization, electrotherapy, thermotherapy, cryotherapy and education. Manual therapy is one method of mobilization and refers to treatment which requires the use of one's hands – aside from applying machinery! Although the definition is broad, manual therapy is a small part of physiotherapy and is only as effective as the ability to accurately detect the dysfunciton for which it is indicated.

The intent of this workbook is to assist the student in acquiring the skills of manual therapy for the vertebral column and pelvic girdle both in examination and treatment techniques by detailed exposition and illustration. The techniques outlined in this workbook are not meant to be exclusive of all others, but are rather a solid base from which the learning therapist can expand. It is hoped that this workbook will be used as an adjunct to the Canadian Orthopaedic Manipulative Therapy courses, part of which requires the instruction of these examination and treatment techniques.

For the beginner, we have purposely presented the techniques in a dissected manner recognising that the skilled clinician may view this dissection as abuse of the art. Indeed, experience teaches us that dogma and recipes have no place in the science or the art of manual therapy, however, for each and everyone of us, there was a beginning.

Diane and Mari, 1985

PREFACE TO THE SECOND EDITION

It has been eleven years since the first edition of this text was published and this decade has seen many changes in manual therapy. While the pendulum appears to be swinging away from 'passive therapy' towards an active approach to spinal care, manual therapy will always be a significant part of total rehabilitation. When joint mechanics are dysfunctional, aggressive and repetitive exercises can lead to overuse syndromes of the soft tissue.

Passive tests remain a necessary component of evaluation as this is our only means of ruling out segmental instabilities, neurological impairment and vascular insufficiencies which, if undiagnosed, may lead to serious consequences. Our techniques have become more refined and in some regions more specific. All areas have been significantly modified since the first edition. These modifications reflect the learning process and represent the work of many physiotherapists internationally. We are indebted to many for sharing their expertise and for allowing us to share it with you. We would like to acknowledge the assistance of our associates without whom this work would not be possible, our models – Pam Simpson, Boyd Glen-Williams, Paul Podgajny, Margaret A. Walsh, our photographers – Roman Sabo and Frank Crymble and our families – Roman, Rónán, Stefan, Tom, Michael and Chelsea.

Diane and Mari, 1996

TABLE OF CONTENTS

CRANIOVERTEBRAL REGION

ASSESSMENT

TREATMENT

MIDCERVICAL

ASSESSMENT

TREATMENT

CERVICOTHORACIC REGION

ASSESSMENT

TREATMENT

THORACIC REGION

    ASSESSMENT

Table of Contents

TREATMENT

PELVIC GIRDLE

ASSESSMENT

Table of Contents

TREATMENT

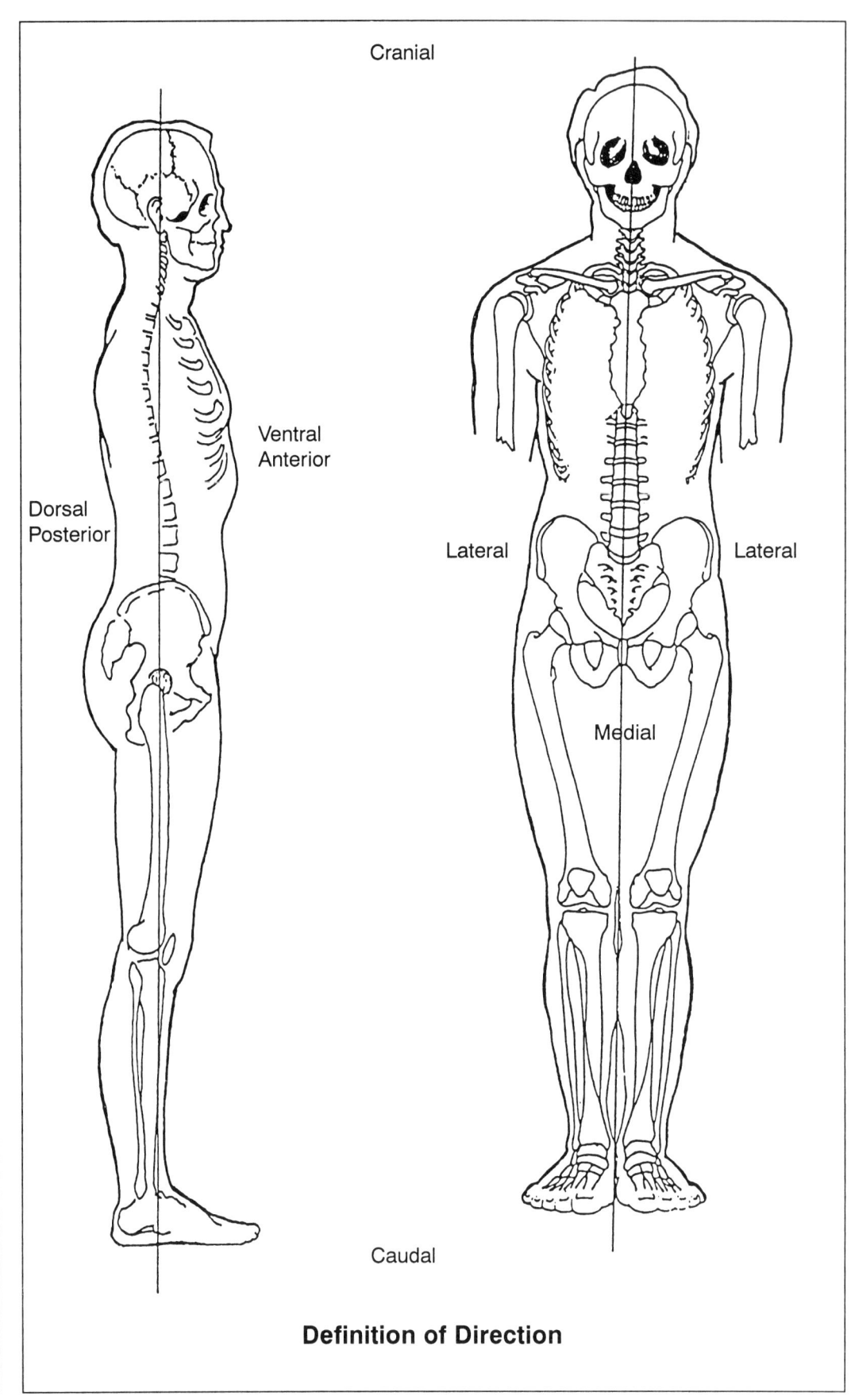

Definition of Direction

Craniovertebral Region

CRANIOVERTEBRAL REGION

ASSESSMENT

CRANIOVERTEBRAL REGION

TREATMENT

POSITIONAL TESTS — OCCIPITOATLANTAL JOINTS

Patient: Sitting.

Therapist: Standing behind the patient.

Palpate: With the index and long finger of both hands, palpate the distance between the transverse processes of the atlas and the mastoid processes of the temporal bones.

Test: a) Flex the joint complex and assess the position of the occiput relative to the atlas by comparing the left with the right side. The side to which the occiput is side flexed in flexion is the side of the shortest distance.

b) Extend the joint complex and assess the position of the occiput relative to the atlas by comparing the left with the right side. The side to which the occiput is sideflexed in extension is the side of the shortest distance.

Addendum: This test may also be performed with the patient supine, but in sitting one can better observe the effect of the weight of the occiput on the joint mechanics.

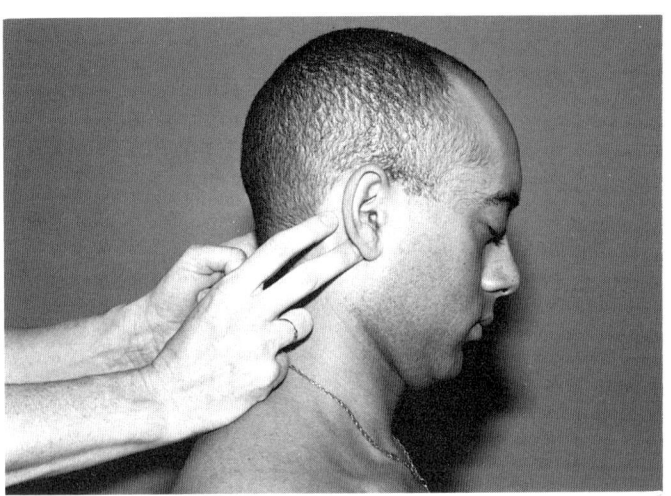

a) Flexion

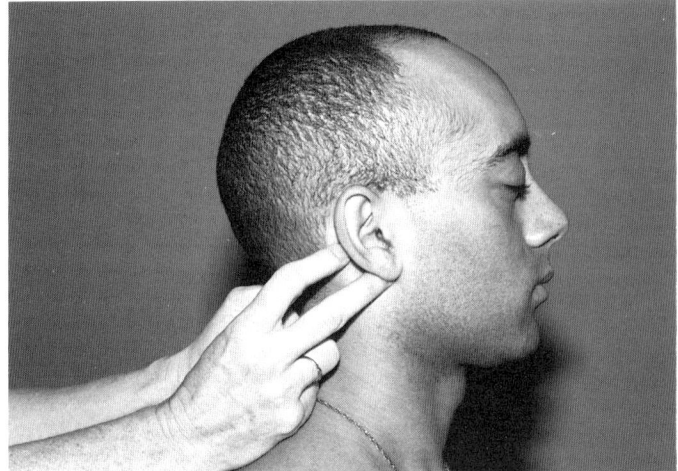

b) Extension

NOTES:

_____

_____

_____

_____

_____

_____

_____

POSITIONAL TESTS — ATLANTOAXIAL JOINTS

Patient: Sitting.

Therapist: Standing behind the patient.

Palpate: With the index and long finger of both hands, palpate the posterior arch of the atlas in the suboccipital gutter and the lamina of the axis bilaterally.

Test: **a)** Flex the joint complex around the appropriate axis and assess the position of the C1 vertebra relative to C2 by noting the position of the posterior arch relative to the corresponding lamina of C2. A dorsal left posterior arch of C1 relative to the left lamina of C2 is indicative of a left rotated position of the C1-2 joint complex in flexion.

b) Extend the joint complex around the appropriate axis and assess the position of the C1 posterior arch relative to the corresponding lamina of C2. A dorsal left posterior arch of C1 relative to the C2 left lamina is indicative of a left rotated position of the C1-2 joint complex in extension.

Addendum: This test may also be performed with the patient supine, but in sitting one can better observe the effect of the weight of the occiput on the joint mechanics.

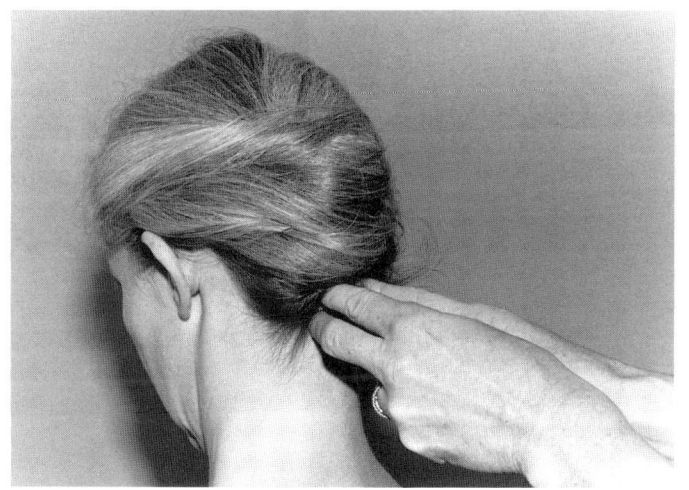

a) Flexion

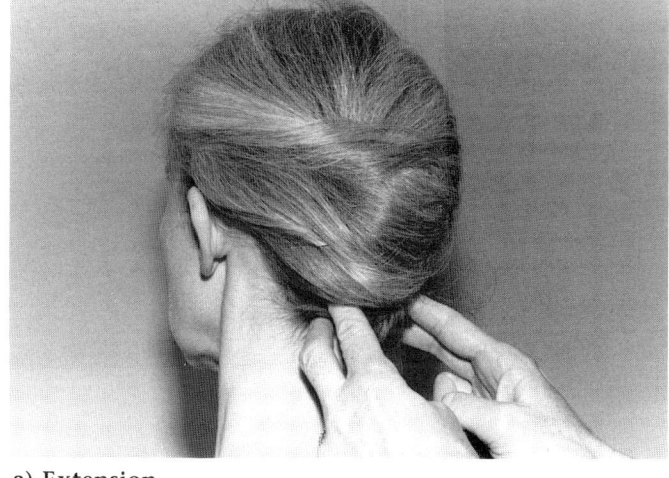

a) Extension

NOTES:

_____

_____

_____

_____

_____

ACTIVE MOBILITY TESTS OF OSTEOKINEMATIC FUNCTION — OCCIPUT, ATLAS

Forward bending

Patient: Sitting.
Therapist: Standing behind the patient.
Palpate: With the index and long finger of both hands, palpate the mastoid processes of the temporal bones and the transverse processes of the atlas.
Test: Instruct the patient to forward bend the head (arrow) around the appropriate axis and note the quantity of motion as well as the symmetry of motion during flexion. The mastoid processes should travel posteriorly along a curved path an equal distance. When interpreting the mobility findings, the position of the joint at the beginning of the test should be correlated with the subsequent mobility noted since alterations in joint mobility may merely be a reflection of an altered starting position.
Addendum: This test may also be performed with the patient supine, but in sitting one can better observe the effect of the weight of the occiput on the joint mechanics.

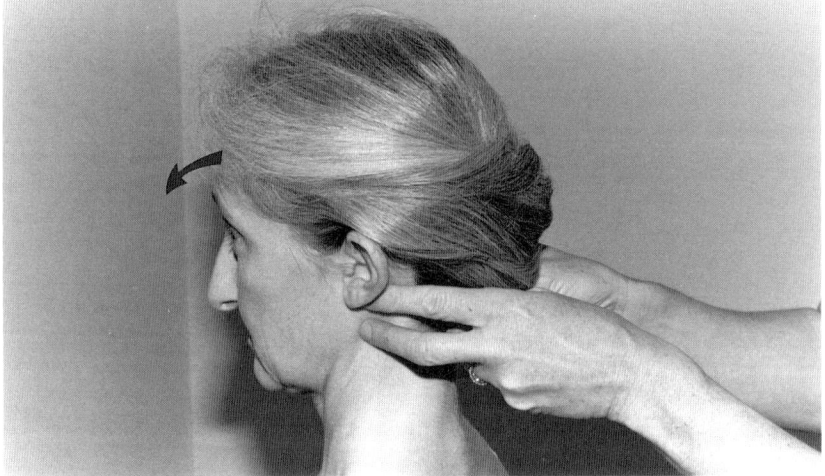

NOTES:

_____

_____

_____

_____

_____

_____

_____

ACTIVE MOBILITY TESTS OF OSTEOKINEMATIC FUNCTION – OCCIPUT, ATLAS

Backward bending

Patient: Sitting.

Therapist: Standing behind the patient.

Palpate: With the index and long finger of both hands, palpate the mastoid processes of the temporal bones and the transverse processes of the atlas.

Test: Instruct the patient to backward bend the head (arrow) around the appropriate axis and note the quantity as well as the symmetry of motion during extension. The mastoid processes should travel anteriorly along a curved path an equal distance. When interpreting the mobility findings, the position of the joint at the beginning of the test should be correlated with the subsequent mobility noted since alterations in joint mobility may merely be a reflection of an altered starting position.

Addendum: This test may also be performed with the patient supine, but in sitting one can better observe the effect of the weight of the occiput on the joint mechanics.

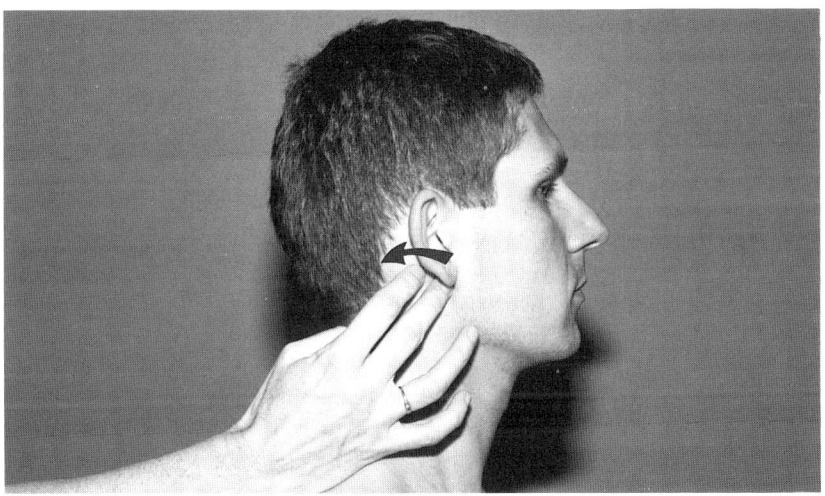

NOTES:

_____

_____

_____

_____

_____

_____

ACTIVE MOBILITY TESTS OF OSTEOKINEMATIC FUNCTION — OCCIPUT, ATLAS

Lateral bending

Patient: Sitting.

Therapist: Standing behind the patient.

Palpate: With the index and long finger of both hands, palpate the mastoid processes of the temporal bones and the transverse processes of the atlas.

Test: Instruct the patient to laterally bend the head (arrow) around the appropriate axis and note the quantity and direction of ease of motion. Conjunct contralateral rotation is usually combined with lateral bending. The mastoid process approximates the ipsilateral transverse process in the coronal plane during lateral bending.
a) Flexion: Repeat the test in flexion of the occipitoatlantal joint and compare the findings.
b) Extension: Repeat the test in extension of the occipitoatlantal joint and compare the findings.

Addendum: This test may also be performed with the patient supine, but in sitting one can better observe the effect of the weight of the occiput on the joint mechanics.

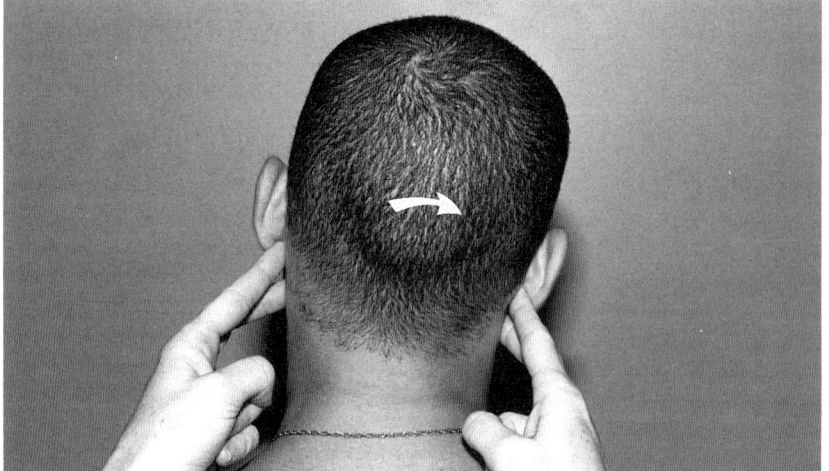

NOTES:

_____

_____

_____

_____

_____

_____

ACTIVE MOBILITY TESTS OF OSTEOKINEMATIC FUNCTION — OCCIPUT, ATLAS

Rotation

Patient: Sitting.

Therapist: Standing behind the patient.

Palpate: With the index and long finger of both hands, palpate the mastoid processes of the temporal bones and the tranverse processes of the atlas.

Test: Instruct the patient to rotate the head (arrow) around the appropriate axis and note the quantity and direction of ease of motion. Rotation is usually combined with contralateral side bending. The mastoid process moves further posterior than the transverse process of the atlas on the side to which rotation is occurring.
a) Flexion: Repeat the test in flexion of the occipitoatlantal joint and compare the findings.
b) Extension: Repeat the test in extension of the occipitoatlantal joint and compare the findings.

Addendum: This test may also be performed with the patient supine, but in sitting one can better observe the effect of the weight of the occiput on the joint mechanics.

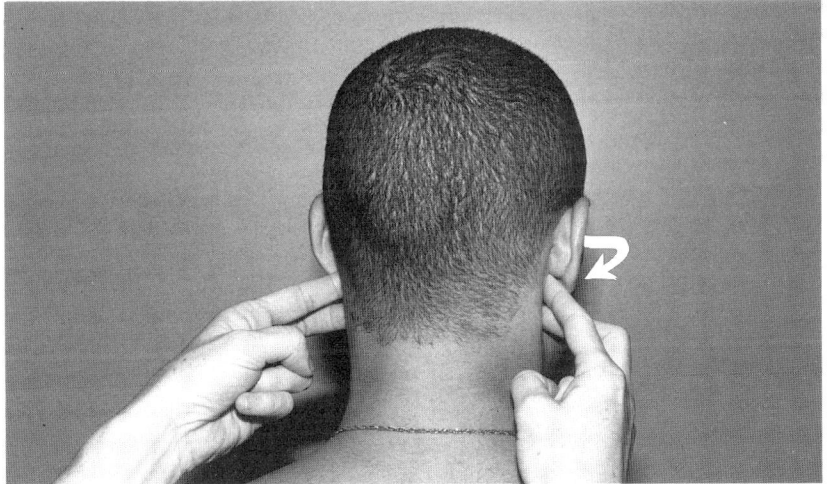

NOTES:

_____

_____

_____

_____

_____

ACTIVE MOBILITY TESTS OF OSTEOKINEMATIC FUNCTION — OCCIPUT, ATLAS, AXIS

Flexion/Extension/Lateral Bending/Rotation

Patient: Sitting.

Therapist: Standing behind the patient.

Palpate: With the thumbs and index fingers, palpate the mastoid processes of the temporal bones and the transverse processes of the atlas. With the long fingers palpate the transverse processes of the axis.

Test: Instruct the patient to flex/extend, and then laterally bend/rotate the head around the appropriate axis. Note the quantity and direction of ease of motion. Palpate any paradoxical movement of the atlas towards the end of the available range, in each motion plane.

Addendum: This test may also be performed with the patient supine, but in sitting one can better observe the effect of the weight of the occiput on the joint mechanics.

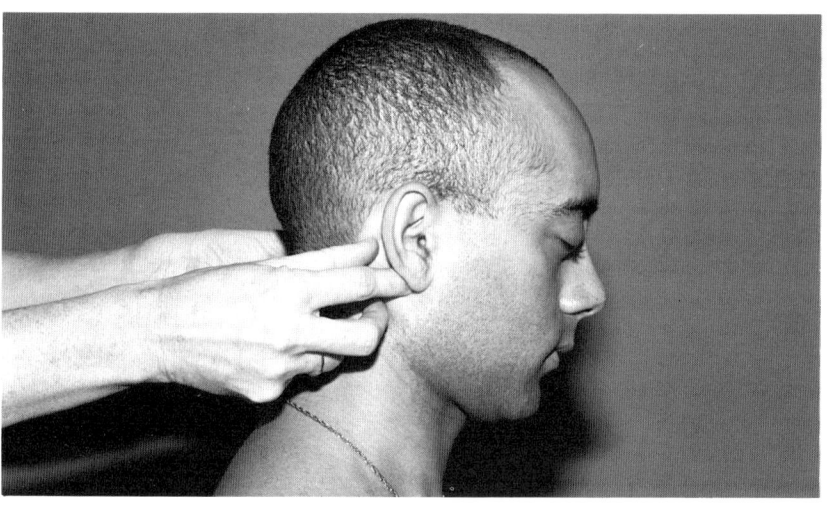

NOTES:

_____

_____

_____

_____

_____

_____

_____

_____

ACTIVE MOBILITY TESTS OF OSTEOKINEMATIC FUNCTION — ATLAS, AXIS

Forward bending

Patient: Sitting.

Therapist: Standing behind the patient.

Palpate: With the index and long finger of both hands, palpate the transverse processes of the atlas and the transverse processes of the axis.

Test: Instruct the patient to forward bend the head (arrow) around the appropriate axis and note the quantity of motion as well as the symmetry of motion during flexion. As the craniovertebral joints are subject to the weight of the head, a paradoxical movement of the atlas may be felt towards the end of the range.

Addendum: This test may also be performed with the patient supine, but in sitting one can better observe the effect of the weight of the occiput on the joint mechanics.

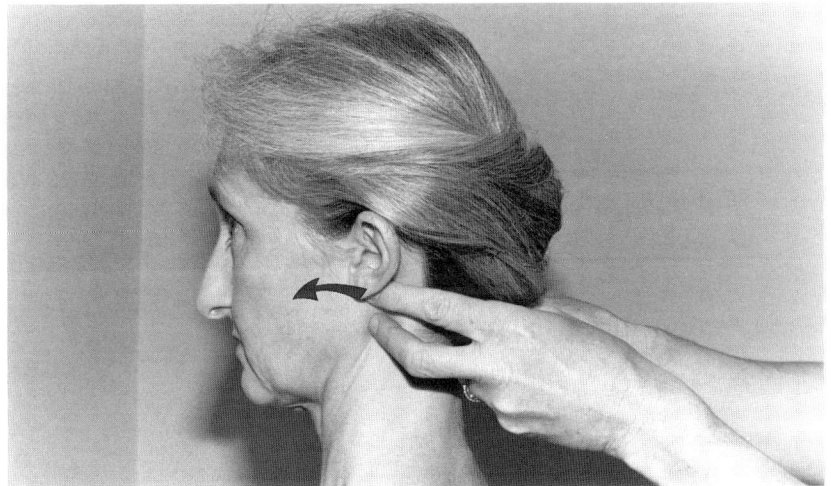

NOTES:

_____

_____

_____

_____

_____

_____

_____

ACTIVE MOBILITY TESTS OF OSTEOKINEMATIC FUNCTION – ATLAS, AXIS

Backward bending

Patient: Sitting.

Therapist: Standing behind the patient.

Palpate: With the index and long finger of both hands, palpate the transverse processes of the atlas and the transverse processes of the axis.

Test: Instruct the patient to backward bend the head (arrow) around the appropriate axis and note the quantity of motion as well as the symmetry of motion during extension. As the craniovertebral joints are subject to the weight of the head, a paradoxical movement of the atlas may be felt towards the end of the range.

Addendum: This test may also be performed with the patient supine, but in sitting one can better observe the effect of the weight of the occiput on the joint mechanics.

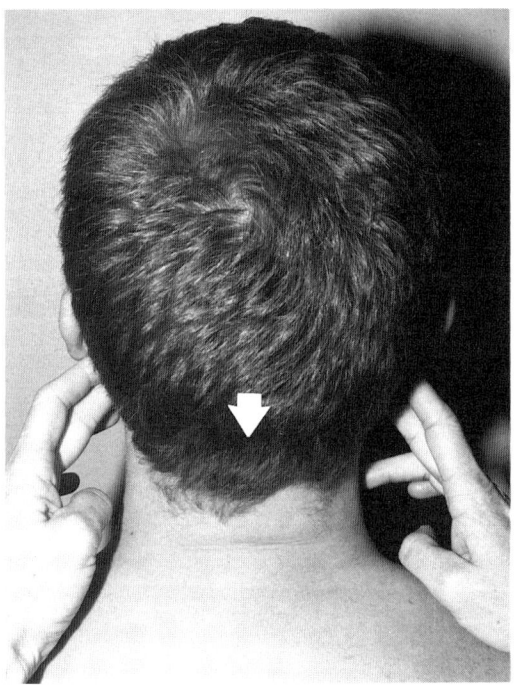

NOTES:

_____

_____

_____

_____

_____

ACTIVE MOBILITY TESTS OF OSTEOKINEMATIC FUNCTION – ATLAS, AXIS

Lateral Bending

Patient:	Sitting.
Therapist:	Standing behind the patient.
Palpate:	With the index and long finger of both hands, palpate the transverse processes of the atlas and the transverse processes of the axis.
Test:	Instruct the patient to laterally bend the head (arrow) around the appropriate axis and note the quantity and direction of ease of motion. As the craniovertebral joints are subject to the weight of the head, a paradoxical movement of the atlas may be felt towards the end of the range.
Addendum:	This test may also be performed with the patient supine, but in sitting one can better observe the effect of the weight of the occiput on the joint mechanics.

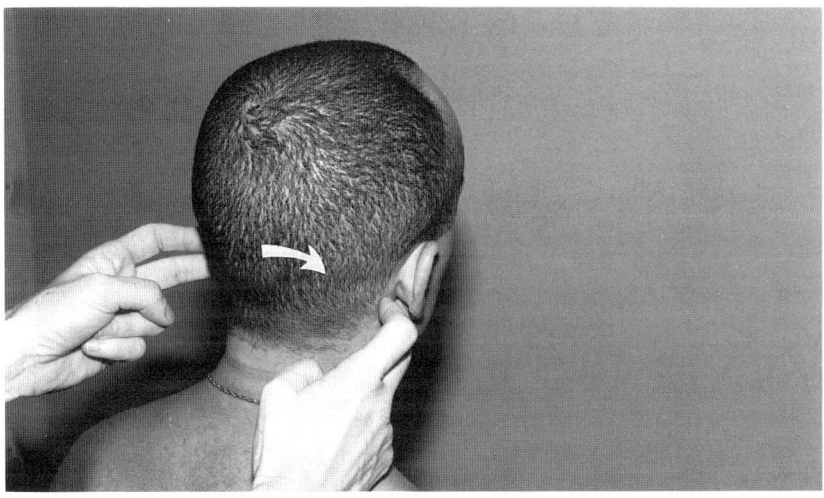

NOTES:

_____

_____

_____

_____

_____

_____

_____

ACTIVE MOBILITY TESTS OF OSTEOKINEMATIC FUNCTION — ATLAS, AXIS

Rotation

Patient: Sitting.
Therapist: Standing behind the patient.
Palpate: With the index and long finger of both hands, palpate the transverse processes of the atlas and the transverse processes of the axis.
Test: Instruct the patient to rotate the head (arrow) and note the quantity and direction of ease of motion. Note any conjunct side bending. As the craniovertebral joints are subject to the weight of the head, a paradoxical movement of the atlas may be felt towards the end of the range.
Addendum: This test may also be performed with the patient supine, but in sitting one can better observe the effect of the weight of the occiput on the joint mechanics.

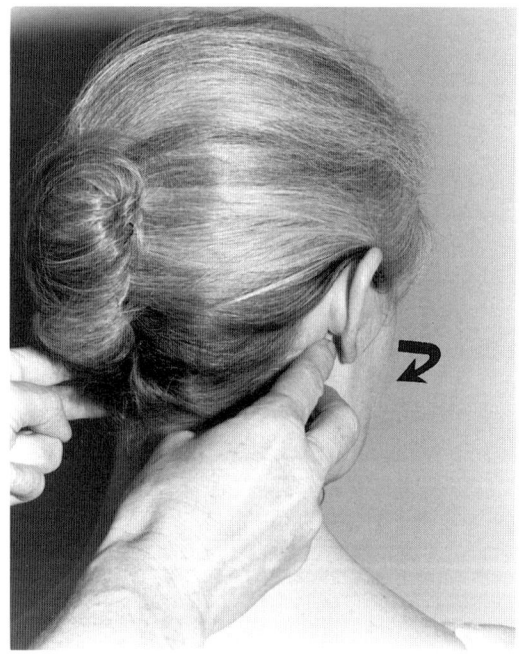

NOTES:

_____

_____

_____

_____

_____

PASSIVE MOBILITY TESTS OF OSTEOKINEMATIC FUNCTION — OCCIPUT, ATLAS, AXIS

Flexion/Extension/Lateral Bending/Rotation

Patient: Sitting.

Therapist: Standing at the patient's side.

Palpate: With the index and long finger of the dorsal hand, papate the occipitoatlantal joints. With the thumb and ring finger of the dorsal hand palpate the lateral atlantoaxial joints. The ulnar border of the fifth finger of the ventral hand is applied to the occiput. Fixation of the cranium should be avoided.

Test: Passively flex, extend, laterally bend, rotate the occipitoatlantal joint around the appropriate axis and with the index and the long finger of the dorsal hand note the quantity, direction of ease, and the end feel of motion at the occipitoatlantal joint. Also note any paradoxical movement of the atlas at the extreme of motion in all planes. With the thumb and ring finger, note the associated movement of the atlantoaxial joints.

Addendum: This test may also be performed with the patient supine, but in sitting one can better observe the effect of the weight of the occiput on the joint mechanics.

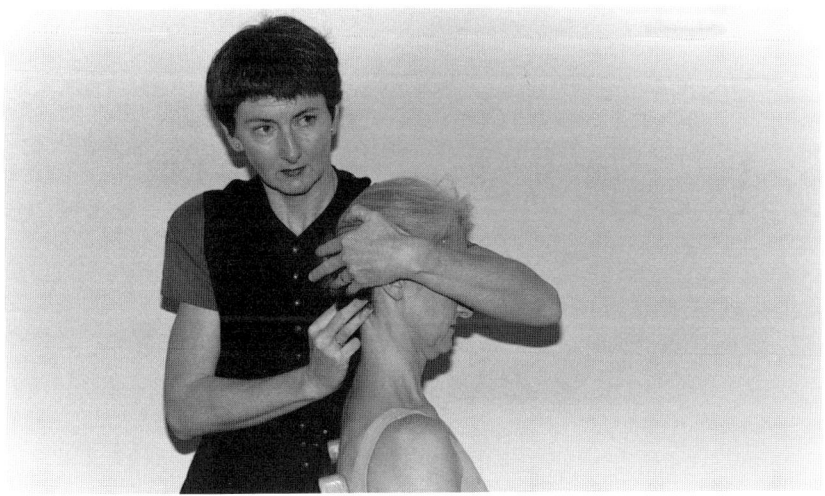

NOTES: _____

_____

_____

_____

_____

_____

PASSIVE MOBILITY TESTS OF OSTEOKINEMATIC FUNCTION – ATLAS, AXIS

Flexion/Extension/Lateral Bending/Rotation

Patient:	Sitting.
Therapist:	Standing at the patient's side.
Palpate:	With the thumb and index finger of the dorsal hand, palpate the lateral atlantoaxial joints. The ulnar border of the fifth finger of the ventral hand is applied to the posterior arch of the atlas. Fixation of the cranium should be avoided.
Test:	Passively flex, extend, laterally bend, rotate the atlantoaxial joints around the appropriate axis and note the quantity, direction of ease and the end feel of motion. Note any paradoxical movement of the atlas during these motions. Also note the conjunct lateral bending of the atlantoaxial joints during rotation.
Addendum:	This test may also be performed with the patient supine, but in sitting one can better observe the effect of the weight of the occiput on the joint mechanics.

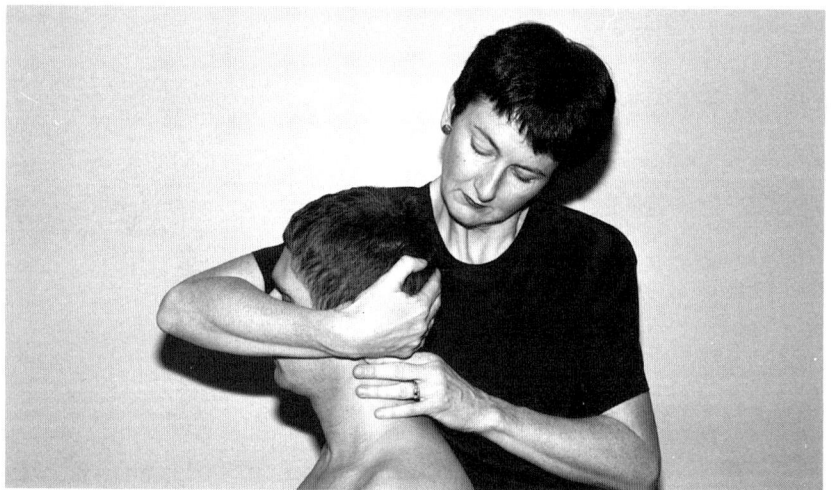

NOTES:

_____

_____

_____

_____

_____

_____

PASSIVE MOBILITY TESTS OF ARTHROKINEMATIC FUNCTION — OCCIPITOATLANTAL JOINTS

Posterior glide right OA – supine

Patient:	Supine, head supported over the edge of the table. The presence of a pillow depends on the flexibility of the cervicothoracic junction.
Therapist:	Standing, supporting the patient's head, facing the shoulders.
Palpate:	With the radial aspect of the index finger, palpate transversely the posterior arch of the atlas. The ulnar border of this hand rests on the table. The other hand cups the occiput while the therapist's shoulder gently supports the anterior aspect of the head.
Test:	Passively left lateral bend and right rotate the occiput on the atlas and apply an anteroposterior force (arrow) to the right occipital condyle in order to produce a glide posteromedially or posterolaterally (depending on the curvature of the superior articular facet of the atlas) over the fixed atlas. Note the quantity, direction of ease and the end feel of motion.

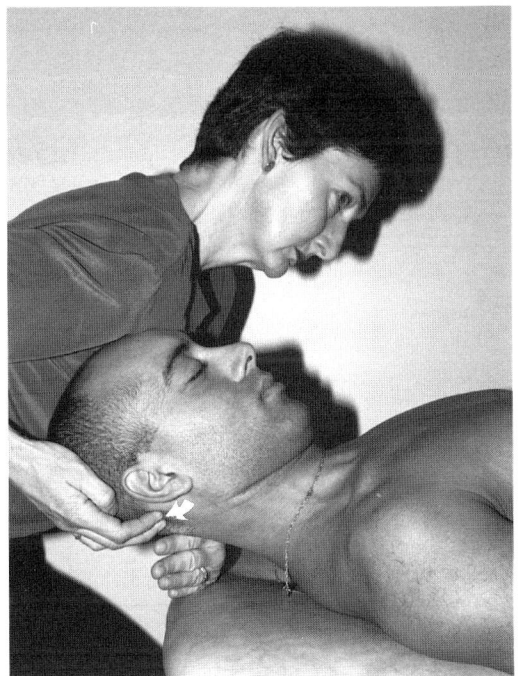

NOTES:

_____

_____

_____

PASSIVE MOBILITY TESTS OF ARTHROKINEMATIC FUNCTION — OCCIPITOATLANTAL JOINTS

Posterior glide right OA – prone

Patient: Prone, head and neck supported in a neutral position.

Therapist: Standing at the patient's side.

Palpate: With the right thumb, palpate the posterior aspect of the right transverse process of the atlas. With the left hand, gently palpate the left aspect of the cranium.

Test: Gently fix the cranium and apply a posteroanterior force to the right transverse process of the atlas with the right thumb to produce a posterior glide of the right OA joint. Note the quantity, direction of ease and the end feel of motion. Repeat the test with the OA joint left laterally bent and right rotated. Note the quantity, direction of ease and the end feel of motion in this position.

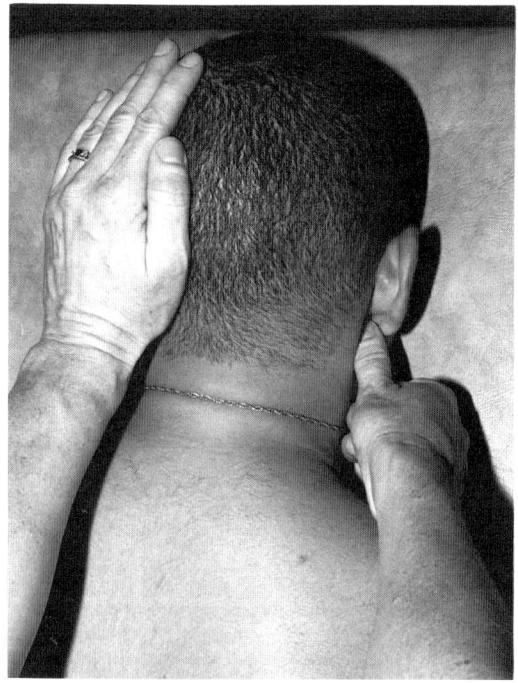

NOTES:

_____

_____

_____

_____

_____

PASSIVE MOBILITY TESTS OF ARTHROKINEMATIC FUNCTION — OCCIPITOATLANTAL JOINTS

Anterior glide right OA

Method A

Patient: Supine, head supported over the edge of the table. The presence of a pillow depends on the flexibility of the cevicothoracic junction.

Therapist: Standing, supporting the patient's head, facing the shoulders.

Palpate: With a lumbrical grip of the index finger and thumb, palpate the transverse processes and posterior arch of the atlas. The ulnar border of this hand rests on the table. With the other hand, cup the occiput and gently support the anterior aspect of the patient's head with the shoulder.

Test: Fix the atlas and apply a posteroanterior force to the right occipital condyle (arrow) to produce an anterior glide of the right OA joint. Repeat the test in varying degrees of right lateral bend/left rotation of the joint complex. Note the quantity, direction of ease and the end feel of motion.

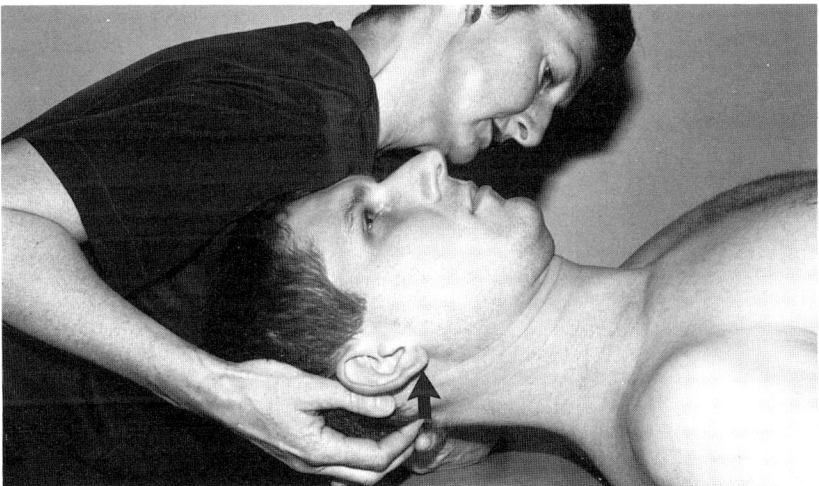

NOTES:

_____

_____

_____

_____

_____

_____

_____

PASSIVE MOBILITY TESTS OF ARTHROKINEMATIC FUNCTION — OCCIPITOATLANTAL JOINTS

Anterior glide right OA

Method B

Patient:	Supine, head supported on a pillow.
Therapist:	Standing at the patient's head facing the shoulders.
Palpate:	With the right thumb, palpate the anterior aspect of the right transverse process of the atlas. The left hand supports the cranium.
Test:	Fix the cranium and apply an anteroposterior force (arrow) to the right transverse process of the atlas to produce an anterior glide of the right OA joint. Repeat the test in varying degrees of right lateral bend/left rotation of the joint complex. Note the quantity, direction of ease and the end feel of motion.

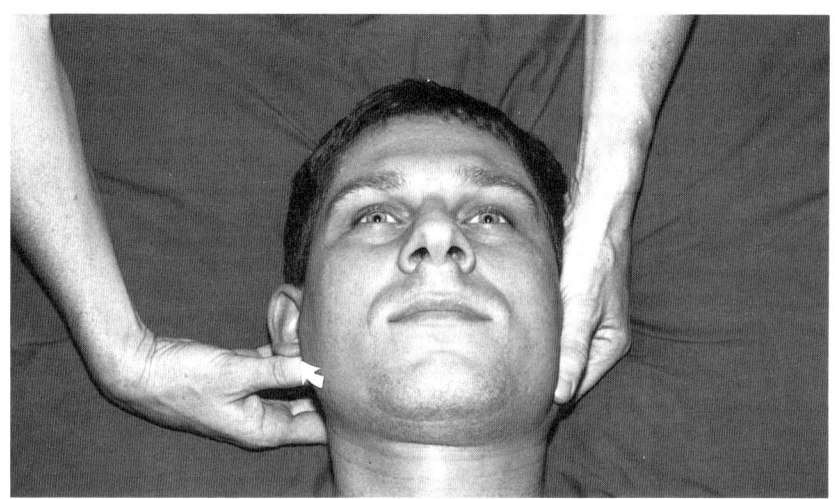

NOTES:

_____

_____

_____

_____

_____

_____

_____

_____

_____

PASSIVE MOBILITY TESTS OF ARTHROKINEMATIC FUNCTION — OCCIPITOATLANTAL JOINTS

Right lateral glide OA

Patient: Supine, head supported on a pillow.

Therapist: Standing at the patient's head facing the shoulders.

Palpate: With the radial border of the MCP joint of the left index finger, palpate the left mastoid process of the temporal bone. With the radial border of the MCP joint of the right index finger palpate the right transverse process of the atlas.

Test: Fix the atlas and apply a force (arrow) to the left mastoid process with the left index finger to produce a right lateral glide of the OA joint complex. Note the quantity, direction of ease and the end feel of motion.

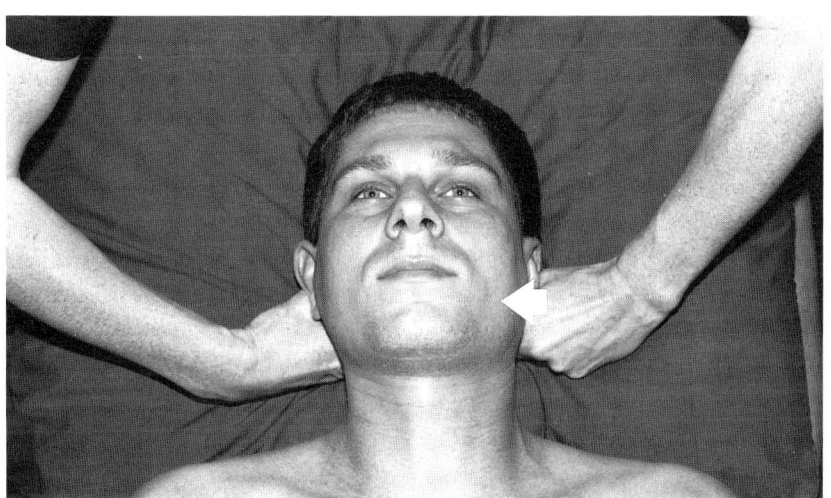

NOTES:

_____

_____

_____

_____

_____

_____

_____

_____

PASSIVE MOBILITY TESTS OF ARTHROKINEMATIC FUNCTION — ATLANTOAXIAL JOINTS

Anterior glide right AA – lateral articulation

Patient: Prone.

Therapist: Standing at the patient's head facing the shoulders.

Palpate: With the left thumb, palpate the posterior aspect of the right transverse process of the atlas. With the right thumb, palpate the posterior aspect of the left transverse process of the axis.

Test: Fix the axis and apply a posteroanterior force (arrow) to the right transverse process of the atlas to produce an anterior glide of the right AA joint. Repeat the test in varying degrees of left rotation of the joint complex. Note the quantity, direction of ease and the end feel of motion.

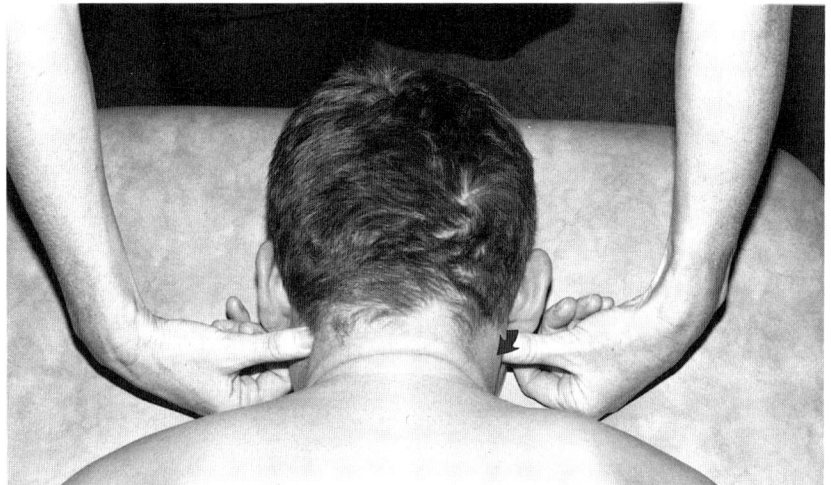

NOTES:

_____

_____

_____

_____

_____

_____

_____

_____

_____

PASSIVE MOBILITY TESTS OF ARTHROKINEMATIC FUNCTION – ATLANTOAXIAL JOINTS

Posterior glide right AA – lateral articulation

Patient:	Supine, head supported on a pillow.
Therapist:	Standing at the patient's head facing the shoulders.
Palpate:	With the left thumb, palpate the anterior aspect of the left transverse process of the axis. With the right thumb, papate the anterior aspect of the right transverse process of the atlas.
Test:	Fix the axis and apply an anteroposterior force (arrow) to the right transverse process of the atlas to produce a posterior glide of the right AA joint. Repeat the test in varying degrees of right rotation of the joint complex. Note the quantity, direction of ease and the end feel of motion.

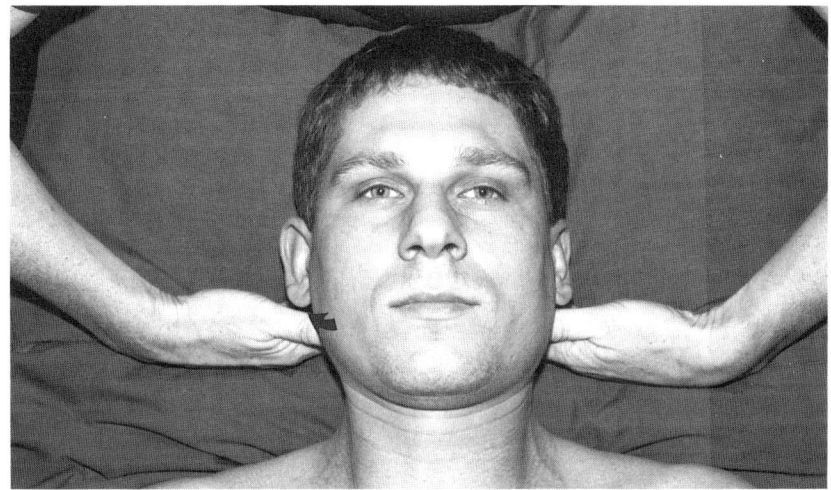

NOTES:

_____

_____

_____

_____

_____

_____

_____

_____

_____

_____

PASSIVE MOBILITY TESTS OF ARTHROKINEMATIC FUNCTION — ATLANTOAXIAL JOINTS

Superior glide – median articulation

Patient:	Supine, head supported on a pillow.
Therapist:	Standing behind the patient's head facing the shoulders.
Palpate:	With a lumbrical grip of the thumb and index finger, palpate the laminae and transverse processes of the axis. With a lumbrical grip of the thumb and index finger of the other hand, palpate the posterior arch of the atlas.
Test:	Fix the axis and apply an inferior force (arrow) to the posterior arch of the atlas to produce a superior glide of the anterior arch of the atlas on the dens. Note the quantity, direction of ease and the end feel of motion.

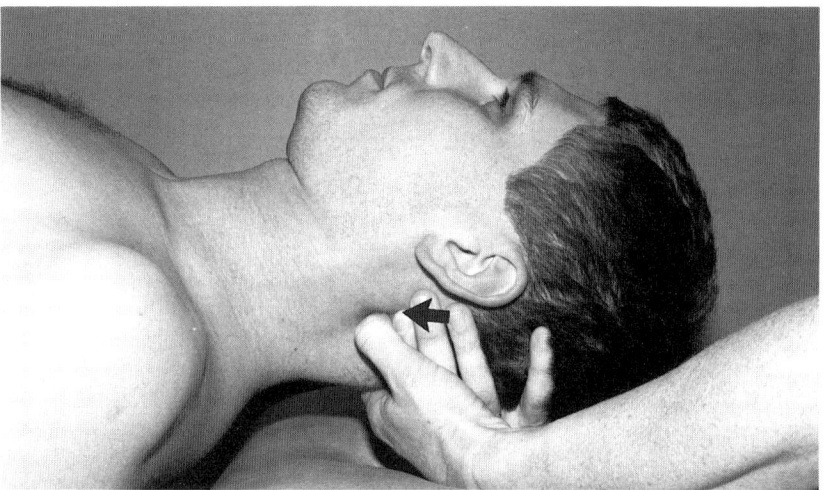

NOTES:

_____

_____

_____

_____

_____

_____

_____

_____

_____

_____

PASSIVE MOBILITY TESTS OF ARTHROKINEMATIC FUNCTION – ATLANTOAXIAL JOINTS

Inferior glide – median articulation

Patient: Supine, head supported on a pillow.
Therapist: Standing at the patient's head facing the shoulders.
Palpate: With a lumbrical grip of the thumb and index finger, papate the laminae and transverse processes of the axis. With a lumbrical grip of the thumb and index finger of the other hand, palpate the posterior arch of the atlas.
Test: Fix the axis and apply a superior force (arrow) to the posterior arch of the atlas to produce an inferior glide of the anterior arch of the atlas on the dens. Note the quantity, direction of ease and the end feel of motion.

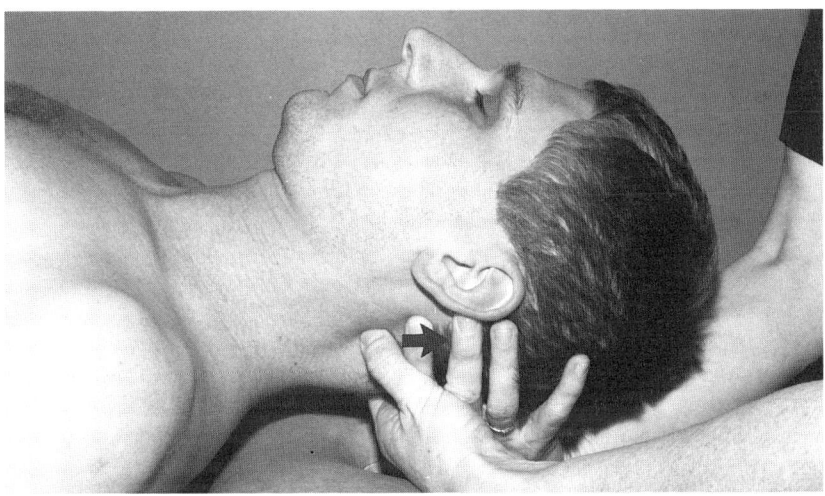

NOTES:

_____

_____

_____

_____

_____

_____

_____

_____

_____

_____

PASSIVE MOBILITY TESTS OF ARTHROKINEMATIC FUNCTION — ATLANTOAXIAL JOINTS

Right lateral glide AA

Patient:	Supine, head supported on a pillow.
Therapist:	Standing at the patient's head facing the shoulders.
Palpate:	With the radial border of the MCP joint of the right index finger, palpate the right transverse process of the axis. With the radial border of the MCP joint of the left index finger, palpate the left transverse process of the atlas.
Test:	Fix the axis and apply a force to the atlas (arrow) to produce a right lateral glide of the AA joint. Note the quantity, direction of ease and the end feel of motion.

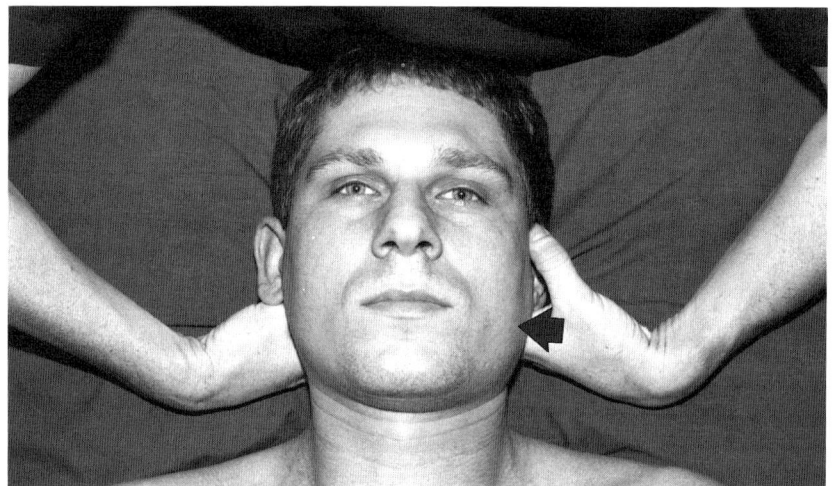

NOTES:

_____

_____

_____

_____

_____

_____

_____

_____

_____

_____

PASSIVE STABILITY TESTS OF ARTHROKINETIC FUNCTION – OCCIPITOATLANTAL JOINTS

OA – posterior translation

Patient: Supine, head supported on a pillow.
Therapist: Standing at the patient's head facing the shoulders.
Palpate: With the palmar aspect of both hands, palpate the sides of the cranium. With the radial border of the index fingers, palpate the posterior arch of the atlas.
Test: Fix the cranium. With the index fingers, apply a posteroanterior force (arrow) to the atlas to produce a posterior translation of the occiput on the atlas. Sustain the force until the end feel is perceived. Note the quantity and, in particular, the end feel of motion.

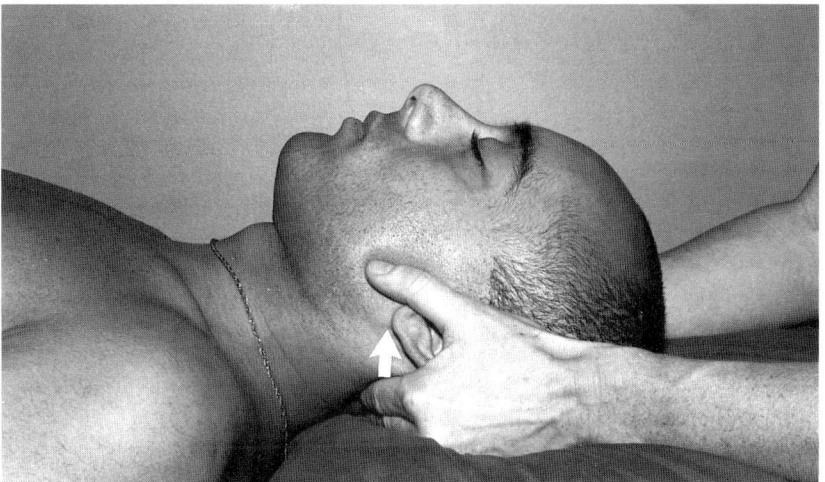

NOTES:

_____

_____

_____

_____

_____

_____

_____

_____

_____

_____

PASSIVE STABILITY TESTS OF ARTHROKINETIC FUNCTION — OCCIPITOATLANTAL JOINTS

OA – anterior translation

Patient:	Supine, head supported on a pillow.
Therapist:	Standing at the patient's head facing the shoulders.
Palpate:	With the palmar aspect of both hands, palpate the sides of the cranium. With the pads of the thumbs, palpate the anterior aspect of the transverse processes of the atlas and axis.
Test:	Fix the atlas and axis and apply a posteroanterior force (arrow) to the cranium to produce anterior translation of the occiput on the atlas. Sustain the force until the end feel is perceived. Note the quantity as well as the end feel of motion.

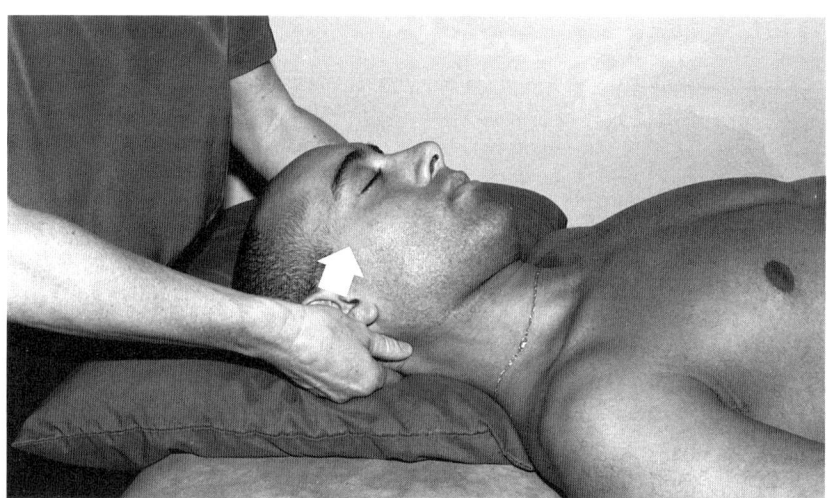

NOTES:

_____

_____

_____

_____

_____

_____

_____

_____

_____

PASSIVE STABILITY TESTS OF ARTHROKINETIC FUNCTION — OCCIPITOATLANTOAXIAL JOINT COMPLEX

Tectorial membrane, articular capsules, OA and AA membranes, alar ligaments, cruciform ligaments

Vertical stability

Patient:	Supine, head supported on a pillow.
Therapist:	Standing at the patient's head facing the shoulders.
Palpate:	With a lumbrical grip of the index finger and thumb, papate the laminae and transverse processes of the axis. With the other hand, cradle the occiput.
Test:	Fix the axis. With the other hand, apply a vertical force (arrow) to the craniovertebral joints through the occiput. Sustain the force until the end feel is perceived. Note the quantity and, in particular, the end feel of motion and the reproduction of any symptoms. Repeat this test **a)** with the occipitoatlantal joint extended and the atlantoaxial joint flexed **b)** with the occipitoatlantal joint extended and the atlantoaxial joint extended. Compare the findings.

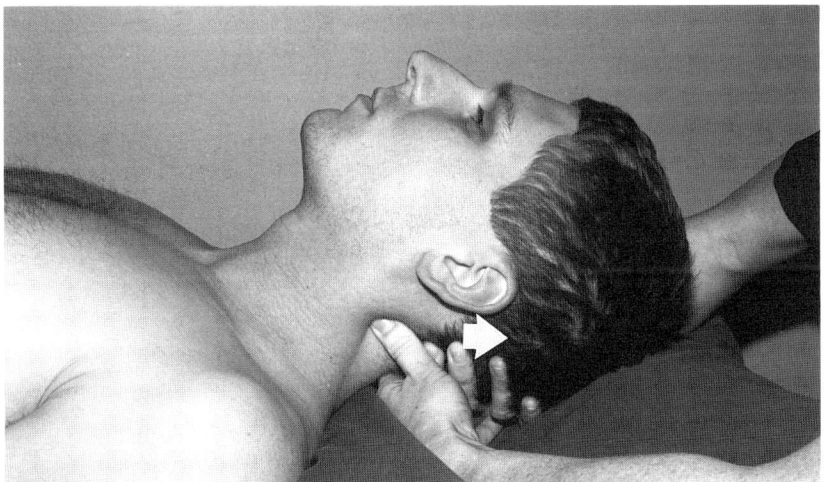

NOTES: _____

_____

_____

_____

PASSIVE STABILITY TESTS OF ARTHROKINETIC FUNCTION — OCCIPITOATLANTOAXIAL JOINT COMPLEX

Alar ligaments – Rotational stability

Method A

Patient:	Sitting.
Therapist:	Standing beside the patient.
Palpate:	With a lumbrical grip of the thumb and index finger, palpate the spinous process of the axis. The ulnar aspect of the fifth finger of the other hand is applied to the cranium with the rest of the hand and arm supporting the head.
Test:	Firmly fix the axis. Using the other hand, left lateral bending of the occiput (arrow) is attempted, thus stressing the right alar ligament. With adequate fixation of the axis, no motion of the head should be possible if the right alar ligament is intact. Repeat the test with the craniovertebral joints in flexion and then extension and compare the findings. The arthrokinetic tests of the occipitoatlantal and atlantoaxial joints must be considered in order to eliminate false positives with this test.

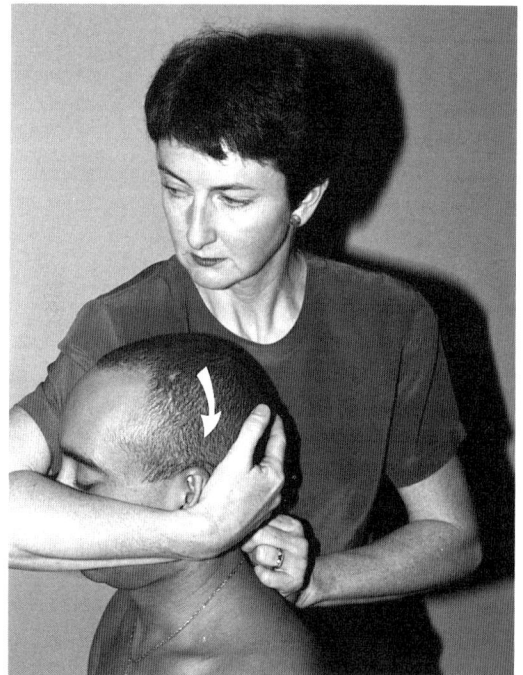

NOTES:

_____

_____

_____

PASSIVE STABILITY TESTS OF ARTHROKINETIC FUNCTION – OCCIPITOATLANTOAXIAL JOINT COMPLEX

Alar ligaments – Rotational stability

Method B

Patient:	Sitting.
Therapist:	Standing beside the patient.
Palpate:	With a lumbrical grip of the thumb and index finger, papate the laminae of the axis. The ulnar aspect of the fifth finger of the other hand is applied to the cranium with the rest of the hand and arm supporting the head.
Test:	Fix the axis. With the other hand, rotate the atlantoaxial joints to the left (arrow). The right alar ligament is stressed during left rotation. Sustain the force until the end feel is perceived. Note the quantity and the end feel of motion. Compare both sides. Repeat the test with the craniovertebral joints in flexion and then extension and compare the findings. The arthrokinetic tests of the occipitoatlantal and atlantoaxial joints must be considered in order to eliminate false positives with this test.

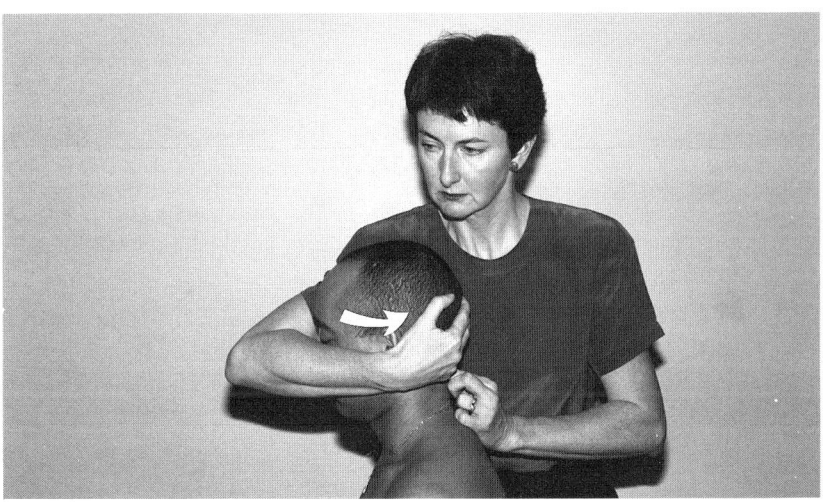

NOTES:

_____

_____

_____

_____

_____

_____

PASSIVE STABILITY TESTS OF ARTHROKINETIC FUNCTION – ATLANTOAXIAL JOINTS

Transverse ligament – posteroanterior stability

Sharp Purser test

Patient: Sitting.
Therapist: Standing beside the patient.
Palpate: With the palmar aspect of the ventral hand, palpate the patient's forehead. With a pinch grip of the thumb and index finger of the dorsal hand, palpate the spinous process of the axis.
Test: Fix the axis and apply an anteroposterior force (arrow) to the patient's forehead to produce a posterior translation of the occiput and atlas on the axis. A clunk may be perceived as the anterior subluxation of the atlas on the axis is reduced. Repeat the test in varying degrees of flexion of the cervical spine.

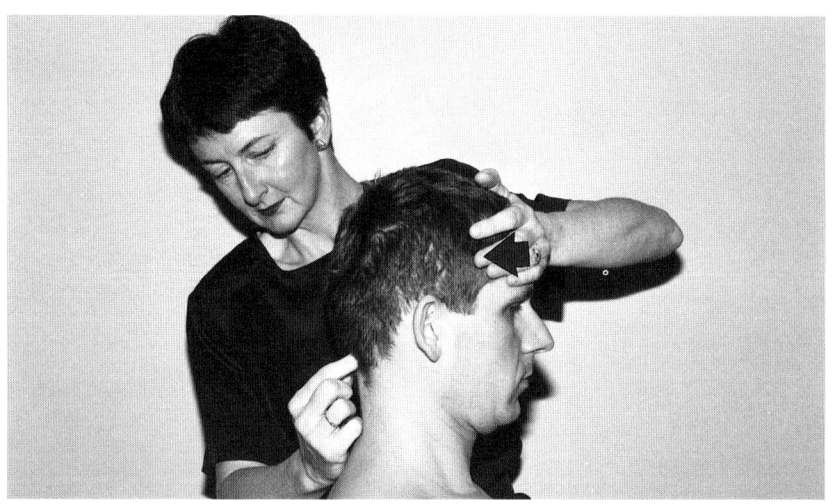

NOTES:
_____
_____
_____
_____
_____
_____
_____
_____
_____

PASSIVE STABILITY TESTS OF ARTHROKINETIC FUNCTION – ATLANTOAXIAL JOINTS

Transverse ligament – posteroanterior stability

Patient:	Supine, head supported on a pillow.
Therapist:	Standing behind the patient's head facing the shoulders.
Palpate:	With both thumbs, palpate the anterior aspect of the transverse processes of the axis. With both index fingers, palpate the posterior arch of the atlas.
Test:	Fix the axis and apply a posteroanterior force (arrow) to the atlas using the index fingers. Sustain the force until the end feel is perceived. Note the quantity and the end feel of motion as well as the reproduction of any symptoms.

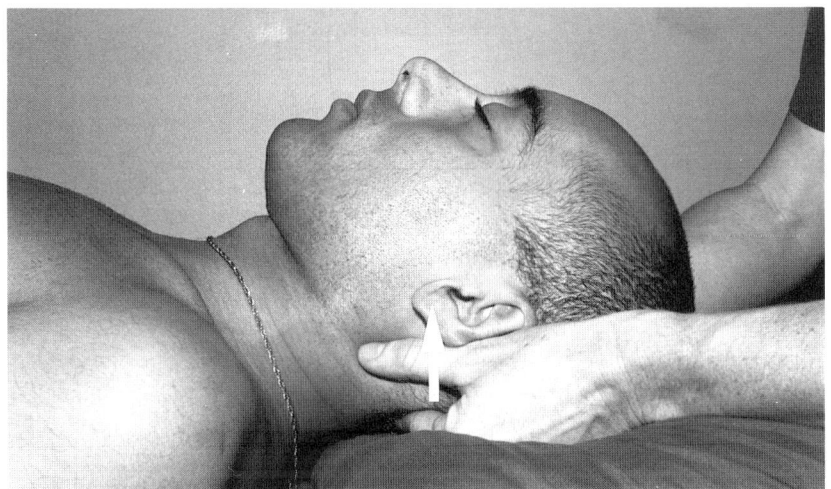

NOTES:

_____

_____

_____

_____

_____

_____

_____

_____

_____

_____

PASSIVE STABILITY TESTS OF ARTHROKINETIC FUNCTION – ATLANTOAXIAL JOINTS

Osteoligamentous ring – right lateral stability

Patient:	Supine, head supported on a pillow.
Therapist:	Standing at the patient's head facing the shoulders.
Palpate:	With the radial border of the MCP joint of the left index finger, palpate the transverse process and posterior arch of the atlas on the left. With the radial border of the MCP joint of the right index finger, palpate the right transverse process and lamina of the axis.
Test:	Fix the axis and apply a right lateral translation force (arrow) to the atlas using the left index finger. Sustain the force until the end feel is perceived. Note the quantity and the end feel of motion as well as the reproduction of any symptoms.

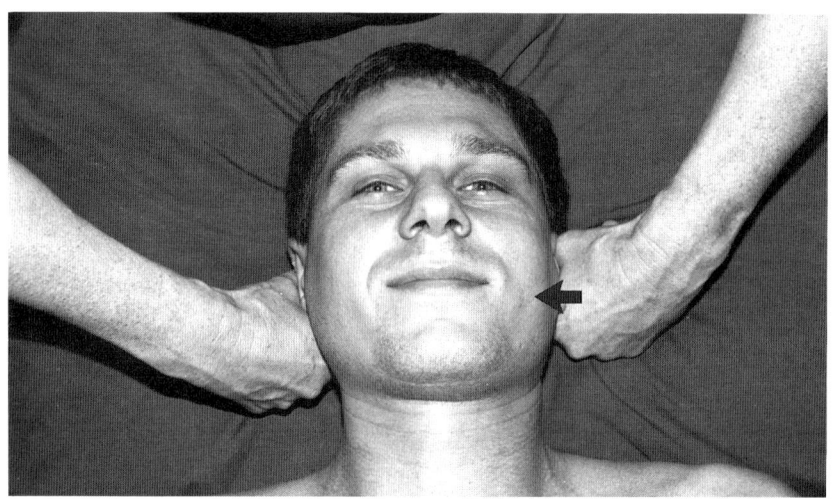

NOTES:

_____

_____

_____

_____

_____

_____

_____

_____

_____

TESTS OF VASCULAR FUNCTION – VERTEBRAL ARTERY

Extension/rotation/traction (lower part of the vertebral arteries C2-C6)

Patient: Supine, head supported over the edge of the table.
Therapist: Standing at the patient's head facing the shoulders.
Palpate: With one hand, palpate the cervicothoracic junction. With the other hand, palpate the cranium and craniovertebral joints.
Test: **a)** Fix the cervicothoracic junction and the craniovertebral region and extend the mid and lower cervical spine (arrow). Hold this position for 30 seconds and note any symptoms or signs produced, especially any cardinal ones (disequilibrium, facial paraesthesia, bilateral or quadrilateral limb paraesthesia, nystagmus).

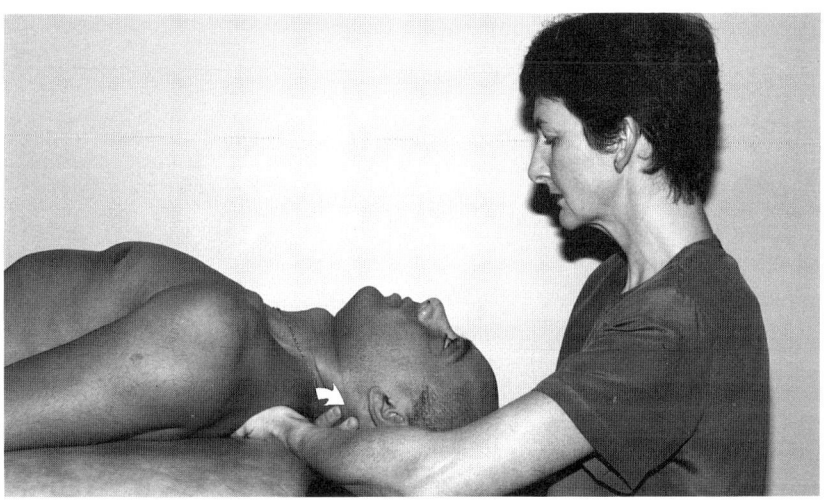

a) Extension of the mid and lower cervical spine.

Continued on page 50

NOTES:

_____

_____

_____

_____

_____

_____

_____

b) From this maximally extended position, rotate the midcervical spine to the left (white arrow), hold this position for 30 seconds and note any symptoms or signs produced, especially any cardinal ones.

c) From this position of extension and left rotation, apply a traction force (black arrow) through the midcervical spine. Hold this position for 30 seconds and note any symptoms or signs produced, especially any cardinal ones.

Repeat these tests with the cervical spine extended, then add right rotation and then add traction. Hold each position for 30 seconds and note any symtoms or signs produced, especially any cardinal ones.

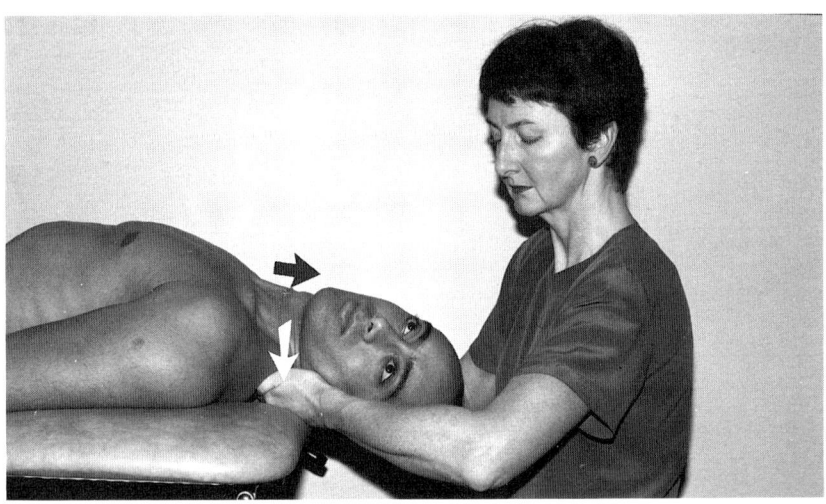

Extension/Rotation/Traction of the midcervical spine.

NOTES:

_____

_____

_____

_____

_____

_____

_____

_____

_____

_____

_____

TESTS OF VASCULAR FUNCTION – VERTEBRAL ARTERY

Craniovertebral extension/compression – upper part of the vertebral arteries

Patient: Supine, without a pillow.
Therapist: Standing at the patient's head facing the shoulders.
Palpate: With one hand, support the mid and lower cervical spine. With the other hand, support the occiput.
Test: a) Maintaining the lower and the midcervical spine in a neutral position, extend the craniovertebral region (arrow). Hold this position for 30 seconds and note any symptoms or signs produced, especially any cardinal ones (disequilibrium, facial paraesthesia, bilateral or quadrilateral limb paraesthesia, or nystagmus).
b) Add a compression force (arrow) through the cranium and hold for 30 seconds. Note the presence of any signs or symptoms, especially any cardinal ones.
c) Rotate the craniovertebral region to the left (arrow). Hold this position for 30 seconds. Note the presence of any signs or symptoms, especially any cardinal ones.

Repeat these tests with the craniovertebral region right rotated and note any signs or symptoms produced, especially any cardinal ones.

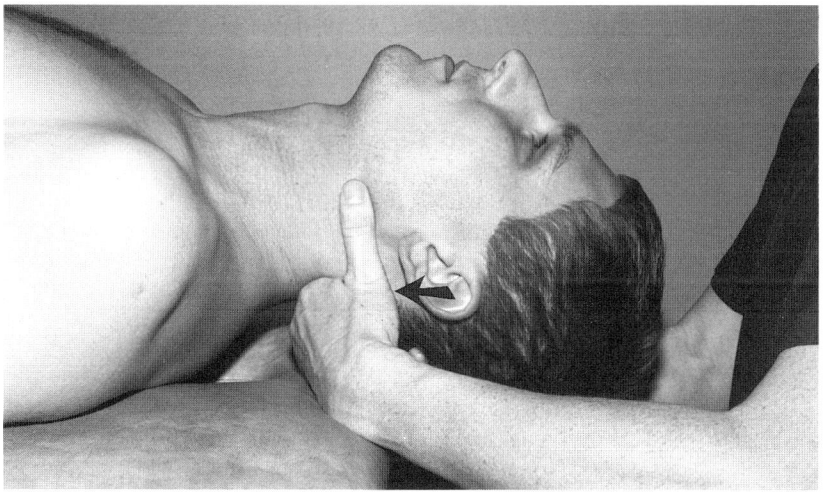

a) Extension of the craniovertebral region.

continued on page 52

NOTES:

_____

_____

_____

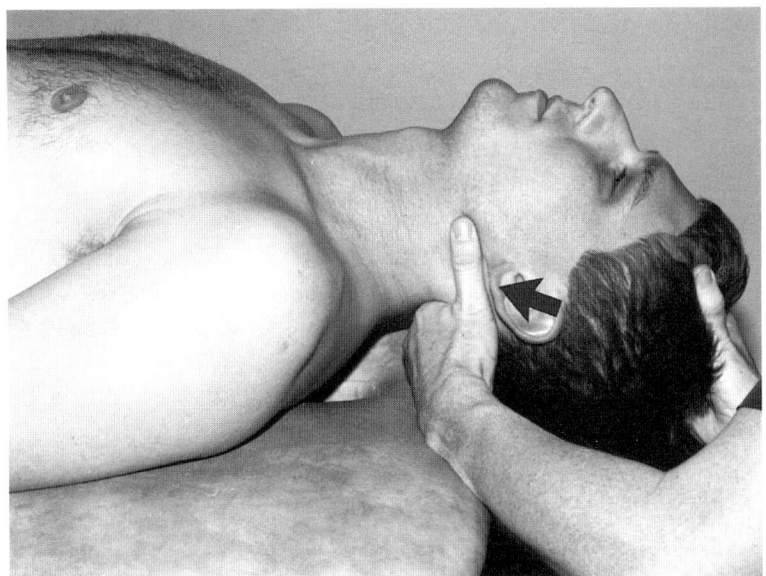

b) Compression of the craniovertebral region.

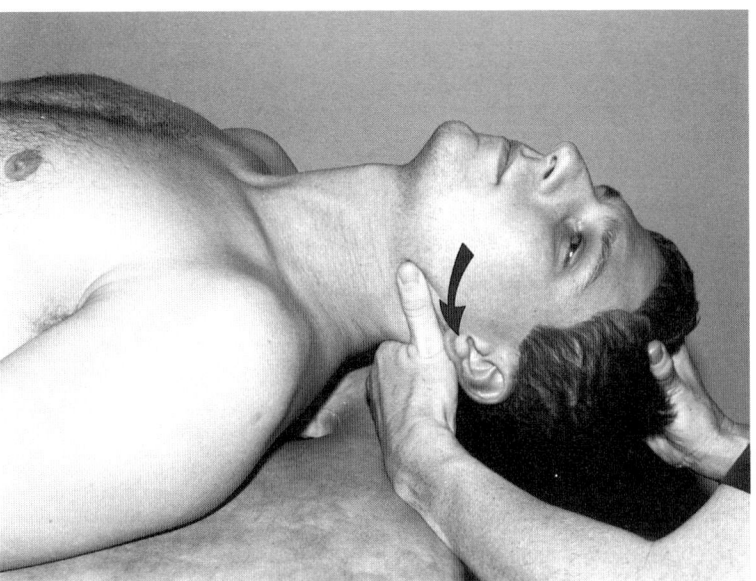

c) Rotation of the craniovertebral region.

NOTES:

_____

_____

_____

_____

_____

_____

_____

TESTS OF VASCULAR FUNCTION – VERTEBRAL ARTERY

Premobilization test for vertebral artery patency

Prior to a grade 1 to 5 passive or active mobilization of the cervical spine, the vertebral artery patency is tested by maintaining the immediate premobilization position for 30 seconds. Note the presence of any signs or symptoms, especially any cardinal ones (disequilibrium, facial paraesthesia, bilateral or quadrilateral limb paraesthesia, or nystagmus).

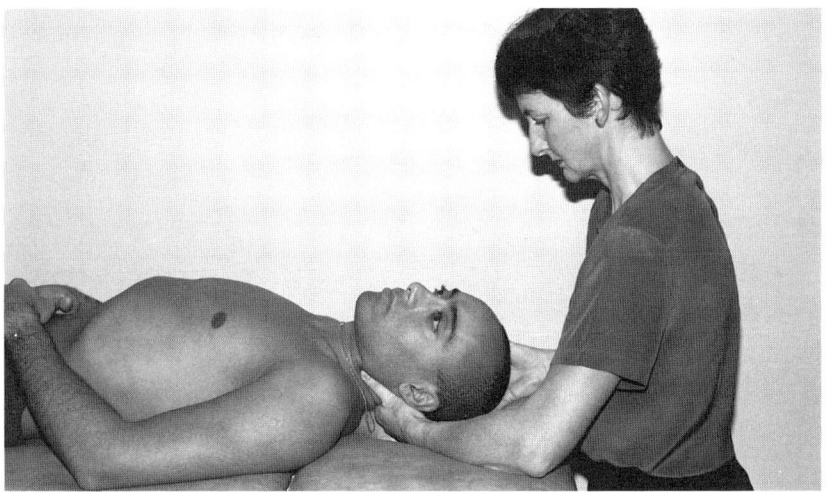

NOTES:

_____

_____

_____

_____

_____

_____

_____

_____

_____

_____

_____

_____

MOBILIZATION TECHNIQUES – OCCIPITOATLANTAL JOINTS

Restriction of flexion (posterior glide) – supine

Patient: Supine, head supported over the edge of the table. The presence of a pillow depends on the flexibility of the cervicothoracic junction.

Therapist: Standing at the patient's head facing the shoulders and supporting the head.

Palpate: With the radial aspect of the MCP joint of the index finger of one hand, palpate transversely the posterior arch of the atlas. The ulnar border of this hand rests on the table. With the other hand, cup the occiput. The patient's forehead is gently supported by the therapist's shoulder.

Localization: Flex the occipitoatlantal joints to the motion barrier with the hand controlling the head.

Mobilization: **Passive** – Apply a grade 1 to 4 anteroposterior force (arrow) to the occiput allowing it to translate on the fixed atlas, thus producing a posterior glide of the occiptoatlantal joints.

Active – From the motion barrier, instruct the patient to gently meet the therapist's resistance. The direction of resistance is that which facilitates further flexion. The isometric contraction is held for up to 5 seconds, and followed by a period of complete relaxation. The joint is then passively taken to the new motion barrier. The technique is repeated 3 times and followed by a re-evaluation of osteokinematic, arthrokinematic and arthrokinetic function.

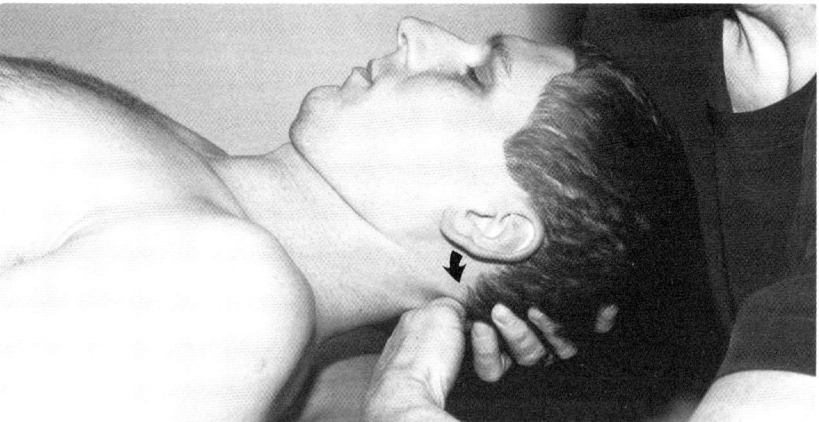

NOTES:

_____

_____

MOBILIZATION TECHNIQUES – OCCIPITOATLANTAL JOINTS

Restriction of flexion (posterior glide) – sitting

Patient: Sitting, spine supported against the chair.

Therapist: Standing at the patient's side.

Palpate: With a lumbrical grip of the index finger and thumb of the dorsal hand, palpate the posterior arch and tranverse processes of the atlas. The other hand and forearm cradles the cranium while supporting the mastoid processes bilaterally.

Localization: With the lower cervical spine in a neutral position, flex the occipitoatlantal joints to the motion barrier.

Mobilization: **Passive** – Fix the atlas and apply a grade 1 to 4 anteroposterior force (arrow) to the occiput, thus posteriorly gliding the occipitoatlantal joints.

Active – From the motion barrier, instruct the patient to gently meet the therapist's resistance. The direction of resistance is that which facilitates further flexion. The isometric contraction is held for up to 5 seconds and folowed by a period of complete relaxation. The joint is then passively taken to the new motion barrier. The technique is repeated 3 times and followed by a re-evaluation of osteokinematic, arthrokinematic and arthrokinetic function.

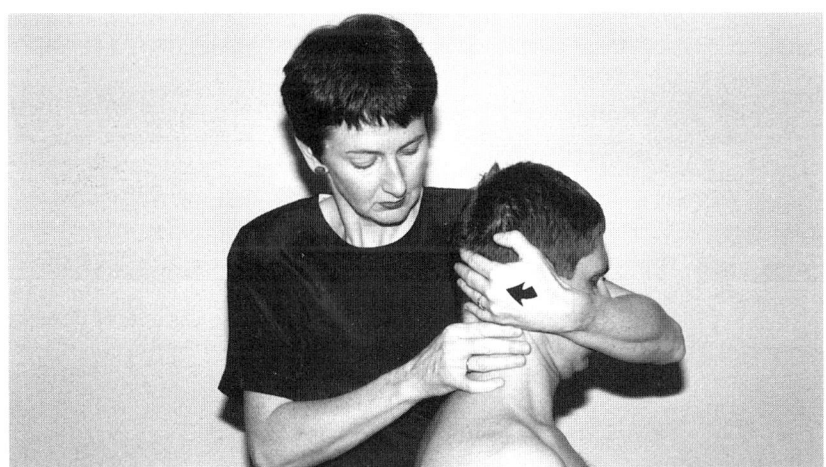

NOTES:

_____

_____

_____

_____

MOBILIZATION TECHNIQUES – OCCIPITOATLANTAL JOINTS

Restriction of flexion, left lateral bending/right rotation (posterior glide – right OA)

Patient:	Supine, head supported on a pillow.
Therapist:	Standing at the patient's head facing the shoulders.
Palpate:	With a lumbrical grip of the index finger and thumb of the left hand, palpate the posterior arch and transverse processes of the atlas. With the radial border of the MCP joint of the right index finger palpate the right mastoid process.
Localization:	The occipitoatlantal joint complex is flexed/left laterally bent and right rotated to the motion barrier.
Mobilization:	**Passive** –Fix the atlas and apply a grade 1 to 5 anteroposterior force to the right mastoid process (arrow), thus producing a posterior glide of the right occipitoatlantal joint.
	Active – From the motion barrier, instruct the patient to meet the therapist's resistance. The direction of resistance is that which facilitates further flexion/left lateral bending/right rotation. The isometric contraction is held for up to 5 seconds and followed by a period of complete relaxation. The joint is then passively taken to the new motion barrier. The technique is repeated 3 times and followed by a re-evaluation of osteokinematic, arthrokinematic and arthrokinetic function.

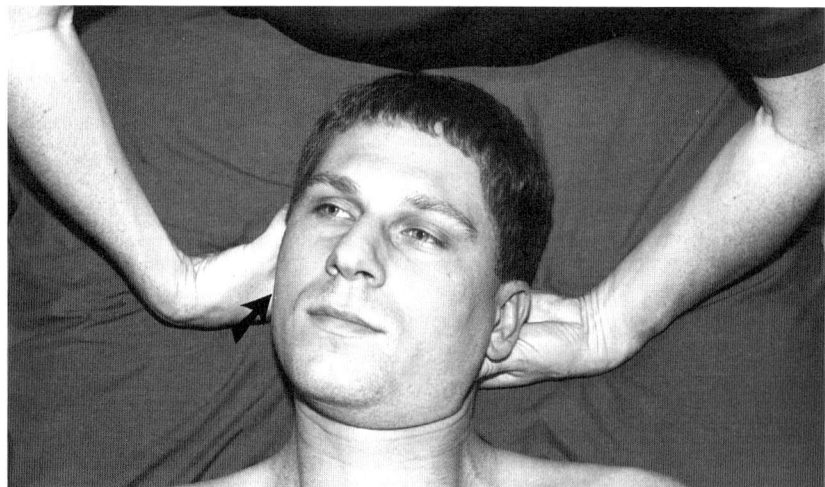

NOTES:

_____

_____

_____

MOBILIZATION TECHNIQUES — OCCIPITOATLANTAL JOINTS

Restriction of extension/right lateral bending/left rotation (anterior glide right OA) – supine

Patient:	Supine, head supported on a pillow.
Therapist:	Standing at the patient's head facing the shoulders.
Palpate:	With a lumbrical grip of the index finger and thumb of the left hand, palpate the posterior arch and transverse processes of the atlas. With the radial border of the MCP joint of the right index finger, palpate the occipital bone medial to the mastoid process.
Localization:	The occipitoatlantal joint complex is extended, right laterally bent and left rotated to the motion barrier.
Mobilization:	**Passive** – Fix the atlas and apply a grade 1 to 5 posteroanterior force (arrow) to the occipital condyle thus producing an anterior glide of the right occipitoatlantal joint.
	Active – From the motion barrier, instruct the patient to meet the therapist's resistance. The direction of resistance is that which facilitates further extension/right lateral bending/left rotation. The isometric contraction is held for up to 5 seconds and followed by a period of complete relaxation. The joint is then passively taken to the new motion barrier. The technique is repeated 3 times and followed by a re-evaluation of osteokinematic, arthrokinematic and athrokinetic function.

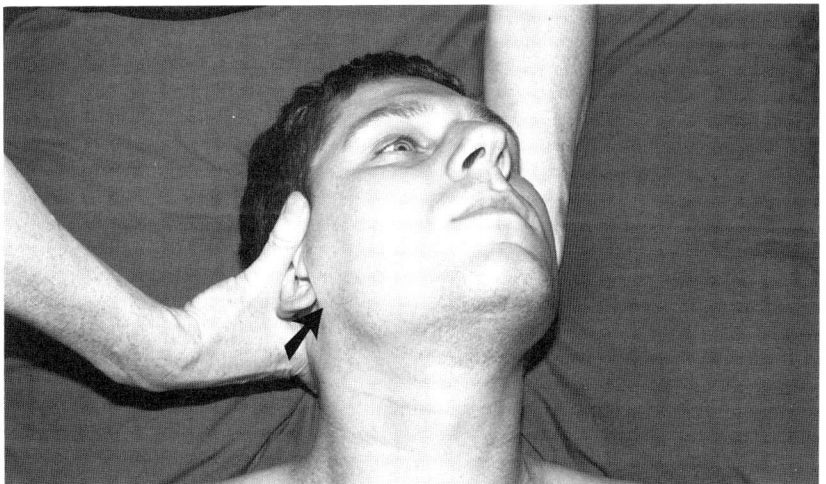

NOTES:

_____

_____

_____

MOBILIZATION TECHNIQUES – OCCIPITOATLANTAL JOINTS

Restriction of extension/right lateral bending/left rotation (anterior glide right OA) – sitting

Patient:	Sitting, spine supported against the chair.
Therapist:	Standing at the patient's side.
Palpate:	With a lumbrical grip of the index finger and thumb of the dorsal hand, palpate the posterior arch of the atlas. With the ulnar border of the fifth finger of the ventral hand, palpate the temporal – occipital region of the cranium.
Localization:	The occipitoatlantal joint complex is extended, right laterally bent and left rotated to the motion barrier.
Mobilization:	**Passive** – Fix the atlas and apply a grade 1 to 4 poteroanterior force (arrow) to the right occipital condyle thus producing an anterior glide of the right occipitoatlantal joint.
	Active – From the motion barrier, instruct the patient to gently meet the therapist's resistance. The direction of resistance is that which facilitates further extension/right lateral bending/left rotation. The isometric contraction is held for up to 5 seconds and followed by a period of complete relaxation. The joint is then passively taken to the new motion barrier. The technique is repeated 3 times and followed by a re-evaluation of osteokinematic, arthrokinematic and arthrokinetic function.

NOTES:
_____

_____

_____

MOBILIZATION TECHNIQUES — OCCIPITOATLANTAL JOINTS

Bilateral distraction

Patient: Supine, head supported on a pillow.

Therapist: Standing at the patient's head facing the shoulders.

Palpate: With a lumbrical grip of the thumb and index finger of one hand, palpate the posterior arch and transverse processes of the atlas. With the other hand, cradle the occiput.

Mobilization: Fix the atlas and apply a grade 1 to 4 traction force (arrow) through the occipitoatlantal joints.

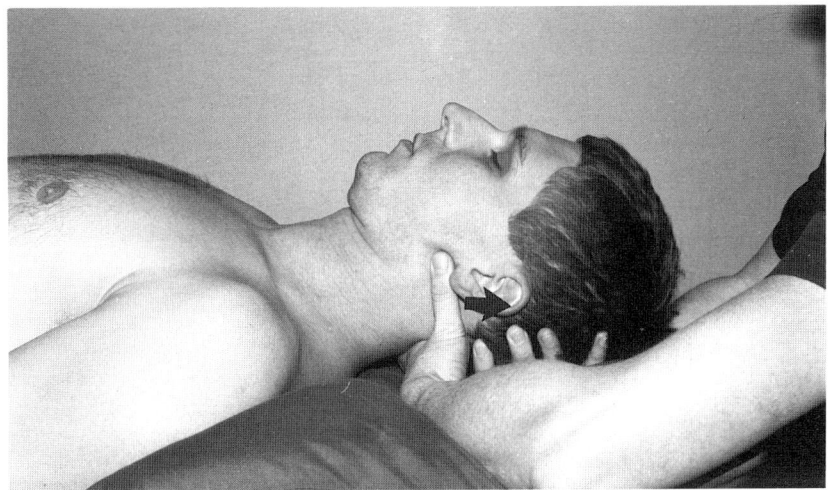

NOTES:

_____

_____

_____

_____

_____

_____

_____

_____

_____

_____

_____

MOBILIZATION TECHNIQUES — OCCIPITOATLANTAL JOINT

Distraction left occipitoatlantal joint

Patient: Supine, head supported on a pillow.

Therapist: Standing at the patient's right side facing the head.

Palpate: With a lumbrical grip of the thumb and index finger of the left hand, palpate the posterior arch and transverse processes of the atlas. With the ulnar border of the MCP joint of the fifth finger of the right hand, palpate the left occipital bone just medial to the mastoid process. The rest of the arm cradles the occiput.

Mobilization: Fix the atlas and apply a grade 1 to 5 distraction force (arrow) to the left occipitoatlantal joint.

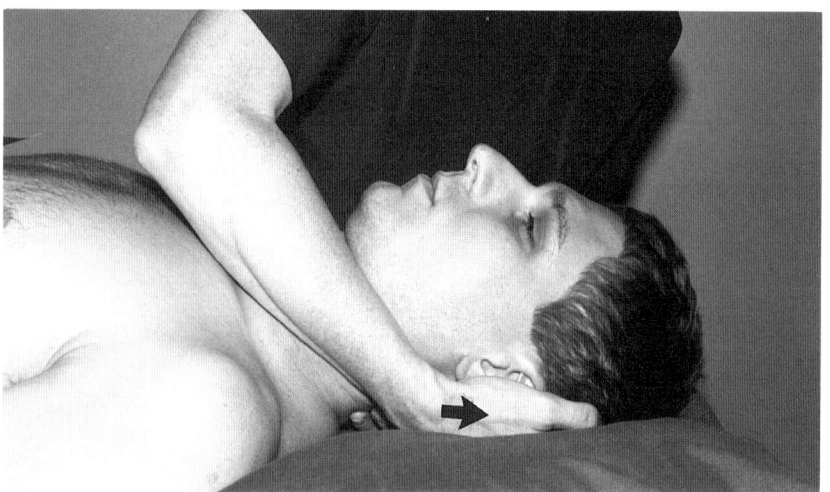

NOTES:

_____

_____

_____

_____

_____

_____

_____

_____

_____

_____

MOBILIZATION TECHNIQUES — ATLANTOAXIAL JOINTS

Bilateral distraction

Patient:	Supine, head supported on a pillow.
Therapist:	Standing at the patient's head facing the shoulders.
Palpate:	With a lumbrical grip of the thumb and index finger, palpate the laminae and transverse processes of the axis. With a lumbrical grip of the thumb and index finger of the other hand, palpate the posterior arch and transverse processes of the atlas.
Localization:	Fix C2 and distract the atlantoaxial joint by applying a vertical force (arrow) to the atlas.
Mobilization:	Apply a grade 1 to 4 traction force to the atlantoaxial joints.

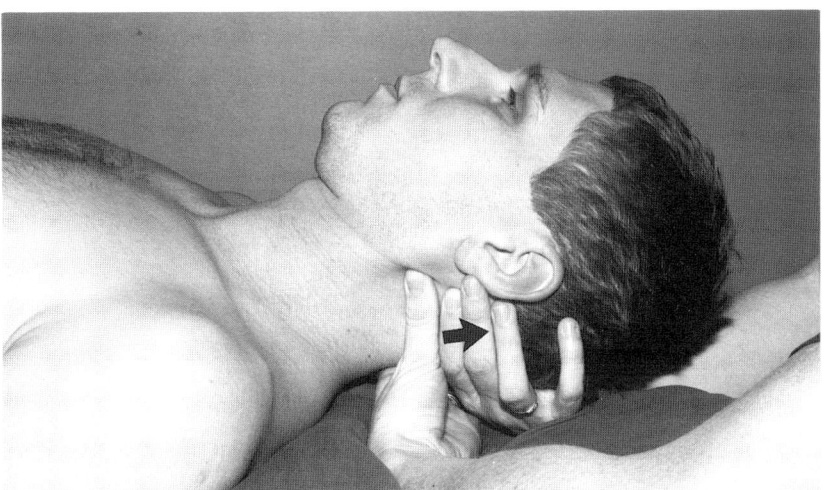

NOTES:

_____

_____

_____

_____

_____

_____

_____

_____

_____

MOBILIZATION TECHNIQUES — ATLANTOAXIAL JOINTS

Restriction of flexion (anterior glide)

Patient: Sitting, spine supported against the chair.

Therapist: Standing at the patient's side.

Palpate: With a lumbrical grip of the index finger and thumb of the dorsal hand, palpate the laminae and the transverse processes of the axis. The ulnar aspect of the fifth finger of the ventral hand palpates the posterior arch of the atlas, the rest of this hand and forearm support the cranium.

Localization: Fix the axis and flex the atlantoaxial joints to the motion barrier.

Mobilization: **Passive** – Apply a grade 1 to 4 posteroanterior force (arrow) to the atlas and cranium, thus producing an anterior glide of the atlantoaxial joints.

Active – From the motion barrier, instruct the patient to meet the therapist's resistance. The direction of resistance is that which facilitates further flexion. The isometric contraction is held for up to 5 seconds and followed by a period of complete relaxation. The joint is then passively taken to the new motion barrier. The technique is repeated 3 times and followed by a re-evaluation of osteokinematic, arthrokinematic and arthrokinetic function.

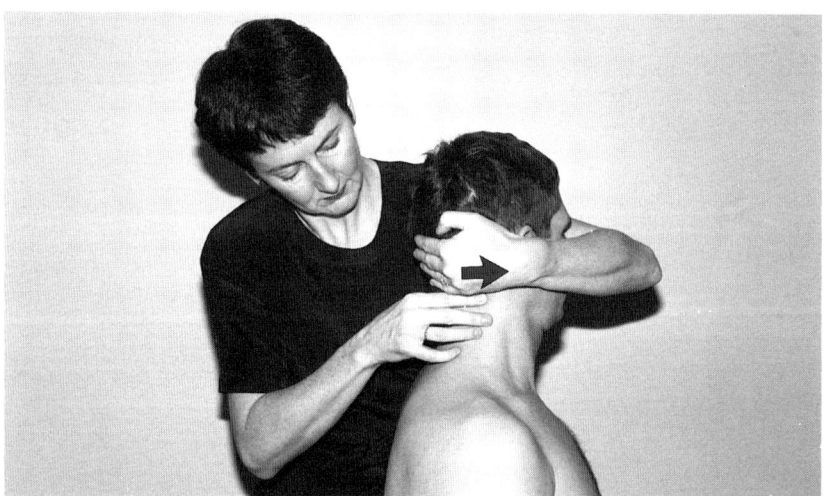

NOTES: _____

_____

_____

_____

MOBILIZATION TECHNIQUES — ATLANTOAXIAL JOINTS

Restriction of extension (posterior glide)

Patient: Sitting, spine supported against the chair.

Therapist: Standing at the patient's side.

Palpate: With a lumbrical grip of the index finger and thumb of the dorsal hand, palpate the laminae and transverse processes of the axis. The ulnar aspect of the fifth finger of the ventral hand is applied to the posterior arch of the atlas, the rest of this hand and forearm support the cranium.

Localization: Fix the axis and extend the atlantoaxial joints to the motion barrier.

Mobilization: **Passive** – Apply a grade 1 to 4 anteroposterior force (arrow) to the atlas and the occiput, thus producing a posterior glide of the atlantoaxial joints.

Active – From the motion barrier, instruct the patient to meet the therapist's resistance. The direction of resistance is that which facilitates further extension. The isometric contraction is held for up to 5 seconds and followed by a period of complete relaxation. The joint is then passively taken to the new motion barrier. The technique is repeated 3 times and followed by a re-evaluation of osteokinematic, arthrokinematic and arthrokinetic function.

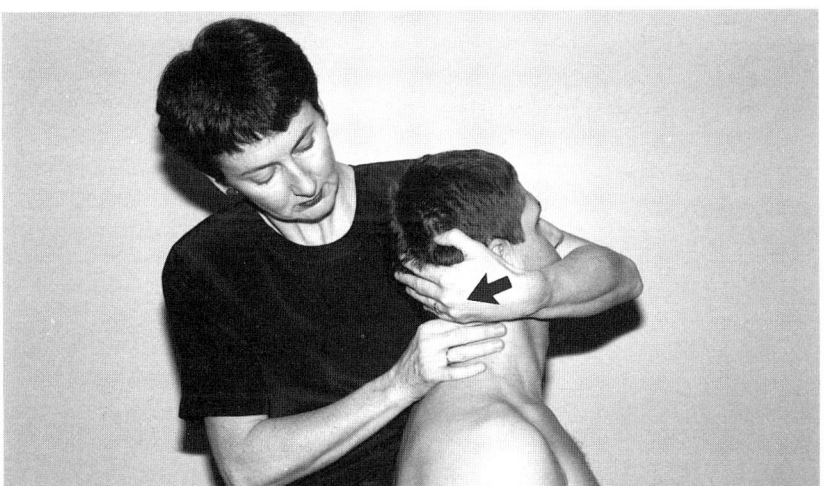

NOTES:

_____

_____

_____

MOBILIZATION TECHNIQUES – ATLANTOAXIAL JOINTS

Restriction of right rotation (posterior glide right AA)

Patient:	Supine, head supported on a pillow.
Therapist:	Standing at the patient's head facing the shoulders.
Palpate:	With a lumbrical grip of the thumb and index finger of the left hand, palpate the laminae and transverse processes of the axis. With the thumb of the right hand, palpate the anterior aspect of the right transverse process of the atlas. The rest of the hand supports the cranium.
Localization:	Fix the axis and rotate the atlas and cranium to the right. Simultaneous left lateral bending of the occiput on the atlas is allowed in order to release the tension of the left alar ligament. Extension of the right atlantoaxial joint facilitates right rotation.
Mobilization:	**Passive** – Apply a grade 1 to 4 anteroposterior force (arrow) to the right transverse process of the atlas thus producing a posterior glide of the right AA joint.
	Active – From the motion barrier, instruct the patient to gently meet the therapist's resistance. The direction of resistance is that which facilitates further right rotation. The isometric contraction is held for up to 5 seconds and followed by a period of complete relaxation. The joint is then passively taken to the new motion barrier. The technique is repeated 3 times and followed by a re-evaluation of osteokinematic, arthrokinematic and arthrokinetic function.

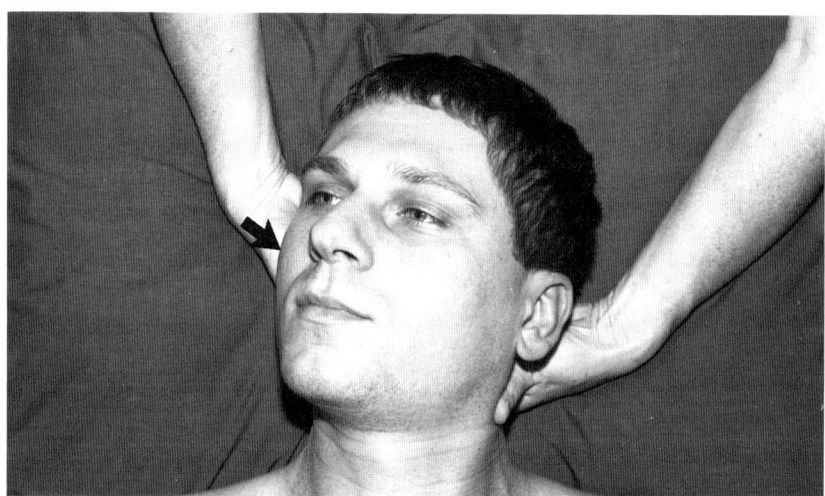

NOTES:

_____

_____

MOBILIZATION TECHNIQUES — ATLANTOAXIAL JOINTS

Restriction of right rotation (anterior glide left AA)

Method A
Patient: Supine, head supported on a pillow.
Therapist: Standing at the patient's head facing the shoulders.
Palpate: With the left hand, palpate the cranium and the left posterior arch of the atlas. With a lumbrical grip of the thumb and index finger of the right hand, palpate the laminae and transverse processes of the axis.
Localization: The midcervical spine, up to and including the C2-3 joint complex, is left laterally bent and right rotated, thus locking the midcervical region. The atlantoaxial joint is then flexed and rotated to the right to the motion barrier. Fix the axis while a posteroanterior force is applied to the left aspect of the posterior arch of the atlas on the axis.
Mobilization: **Passive** – Apply a grade 1 to 5 posteroanterior force (arrow) to the left aspect of the posterior arch of the atlas thus producing an anterior glide of the left atlantoaxial joint.
Active – From the motion barrier, instruct the patient to gently meet the therapist's resistance. The direction of resistance is that which facilitates further right rotation. The isometric contraction is held for up to 5 seconds and followed by a period of complete relaxation. The joint is then passively taken to the new motion barrier. The technique is repeated 3 times and followed by a re-evaluation of osteokinematic, arthrokinematic and arthrokinetic function.

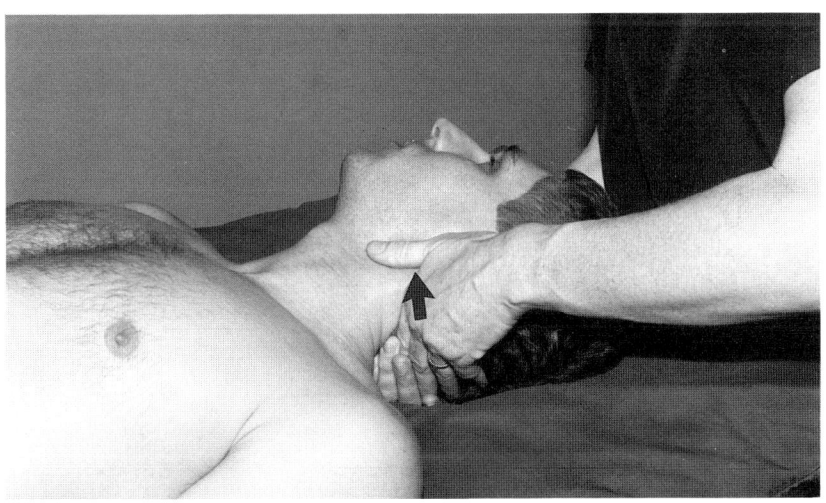

MOBILIZATION TECHNIQUES – ATLANTOAXIAL JOINTS

Restriction of right rotation (anterior glide left AA)

Method B
Patient: Supine, head supported on a pillow.
Therapist: Standing at the patient's head facing the shoulders.
Palpate: With the MCP joint of the left index finger, palpate the left lamina and spinous process of the axis. The other hand supports the cranium and the posterior arch of the atlas bilaterally.
Localization: The midcervical spine, up to and including the C2-3 joint complex, is left laterally bent and right rotated, thus locking the midcervical region. The atlantoaxial joint is then extended and rotated to the right to the motion barrier. A posteromedial force is applied to the left lamina of the axis.
Mobilization: **Passive** – Apply a grade 1 to 5 posteromedial force (arrow) to the left lamina and spinous process of the axis while simultaneously rotating the cranium and atlas to the right. This produces an anterior glide of the left atlantoaxial joint.

Active – From the motion barrier, instruct the patient to gently meet the therapist's resistance. The direction of resistance is that which facilitates further right rotation. The isometric contraction is held for up to 5 seconds and followed by a period of complete relaxation. The joint is then passively taken to the new motion barrier. The technique is repeated 3 times and followed by a re-evaluation of osteokinematic, arthrokinematic and arthrokinetic function.

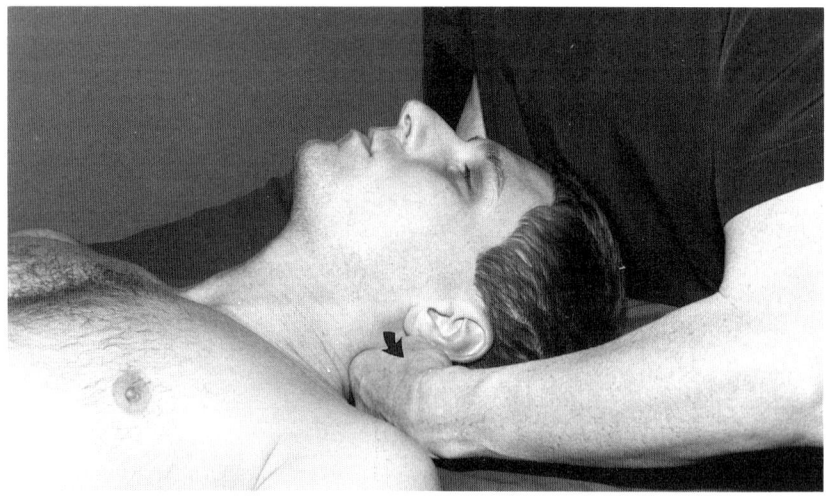

MOBILIZATION TECHNIQUES — ATLANTOAXIAL JOINTS

Restriction of right lateral bending

Patient:	Sitting, spine supported against the chair.
Therapist:	Standing at the patient's side.
Palpate:	With a lumbrical grip of the thumb and index finger of the dorsal hand, palpate the laminae and spinous process of the axis. The ulnar border of the fifth finger of the ventral hand is applied to the posterior arch of the atlas. The rest of this hand cradles the cranium.
Localization:	The midcervical spine, up to and including the C2-3 joint complex, is right laterally bent and left rotated, thus locking the midcervical region. Fix the axis and right laterally bend/rotate the atlantoaxial joint to the motion barrier.
Mobilization:	**Passive** – Apply a grade 1 to 4 right lateral bending/rotation force (arrow) to the atlantoaxial joint.
	Active – From the motion barrier, instruct the patient to gently meet the therapist's resistance. The direction of resistance is that which facilitates further right lateral bending. The isometric contraction is held for up to 5 seconds and followed by a period of complete relaxation. The joint is then passively taken to the new motion barrier. The technique is repeated 3 times and followed by a re-evaluation of osteokinematic, arthrokinematic and arthrokinetic function.

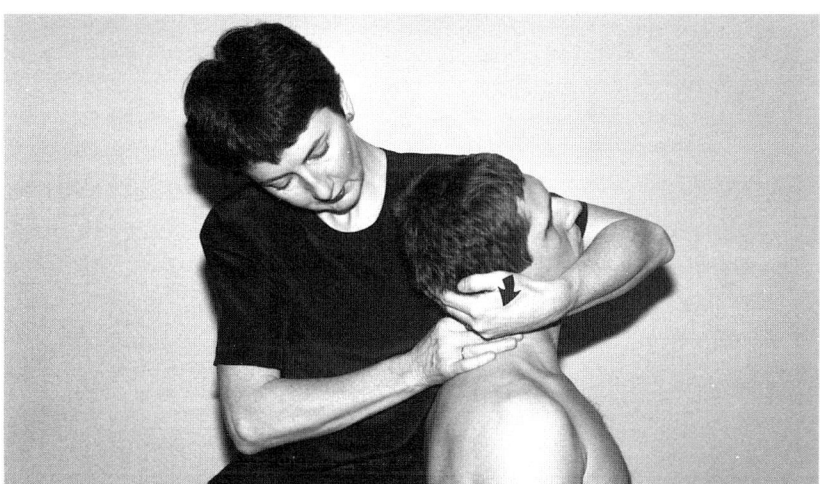

NOTES: _____

_____

_____

MOBILIZATION TECHNIQUES — SOFT TISSUE

Restriction of longitudinal mobility – Suboccipital soft tissue

Patient: Supine, head supported on a pillow.

Therapist: Standing or sitting at the patient's head facing the shoulders.

Palpate: With the forearms supinated and the fingers flexed in a lumbrical grip, palpate the suboccipital tissue bilaterally. The distal 1/3 of the forearms should be supported on the table.

Mobilization: **Do not** use the finger flexors. This produces a digging sensation as opposed to an effective stretch. Apply a slow, steady stretch (arrow) via elbow flexion/shoulder extension and release.

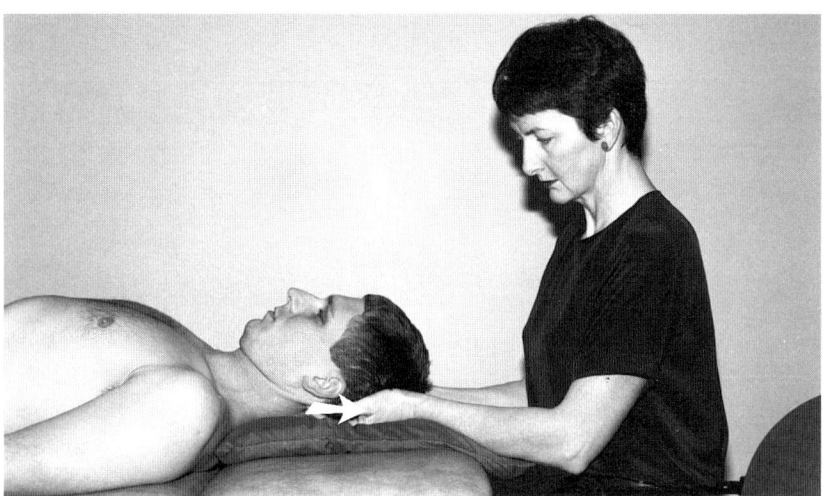

NOTES:

_____

_____

_____

_____

_____

_____

_____

_____

_____

_____

MOBILIZATION TECHNIQUES — SOFT TISSUE

Restriction of transverse mobility – Suboccipital soft tissue

Patient: Supine, head supported on a pillow.

Therapist: Standing at the side of the table level with the patient's cranium.

Palpate: Place the dorsal aspect of one hand against the patient's zygoma. With the index and long finger of the other hand, palpate the posterior arch of the atlas on the opposite side.

Mobilization: Fix the cranium and apply a slow, steady transverse stretch to the suboccipital tissue by pulling the atlas ventrally and medially (arrow). This technique may also be used to enhance rotation at the atlantoaxial joint.

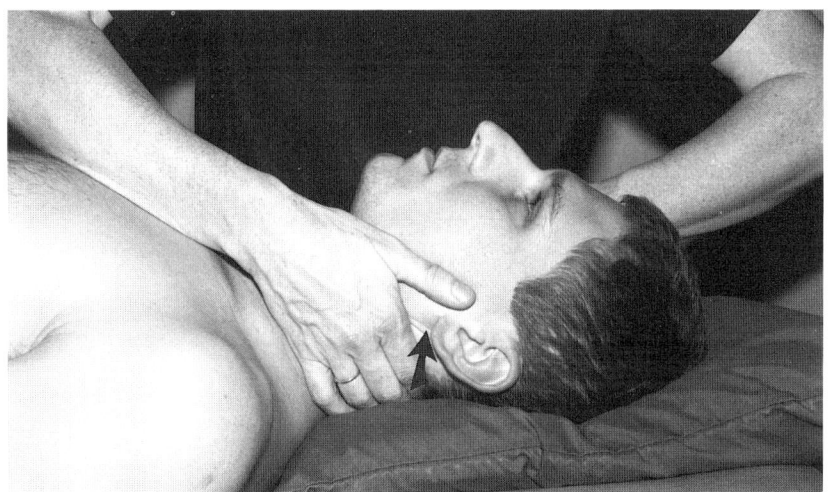

NOTES:

_____

_____

_____

_____

_____

_____

_____

_____

_____

Midcervical Region

**MIDCERVICAL
REGION**

MIDCERVICAL

ASSESSMENT

POSITIONAL TESTS

Patient: Sitting.

Therapist: Standing behind the patient.

Palpate: With the thumbs, palpate the articular pillars of the C4 vertebra.

Test: **a)** Flex the joint complex and assess the position of C4 relative to C5 by noting which articular pillar is the most dorsal. A dorsal left articular pillar of C4 relative to C5 is indicative of a left rotated position of the C4-5 joint complex in flexion.

        b) Extend the joint complex and assess the position of the C4 vertebra relative to C5 by noting which articular pillar is the most dorsal. A dorsal left articular pillar of C4 relative to C5 is indicative of a left rotated position of the C4-5 joint complex in extension.

Addendum: This test may also be performed with the patient supine, but in sitting one can better observe the effect of the weight of the occiput on the joint mechanics.

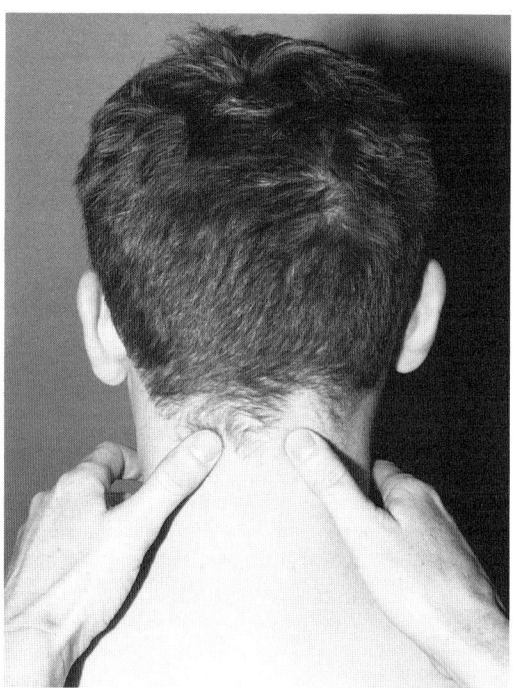

NOTES:

_____

_____

_____

_____

ACTIVE MOBILITY TESTS OF OSTEOKINEMATIC FUNCTION

Forward bending

Patient: Sitting.

Therapist: Standing behind the patient.

Palpate: With the thumbs of both hands, palpate the interlaminar spaces of the two adjacent vertebrae.

Test: Instruct the patient to forward bend the head and neck (arrow) and note the quantity of motion as well as the symmetry of motion during flexion. When interpreting the mobility findings, the position of the joint at the beginning of the test should be correlated with the subsequent mobility noted since alterations in joint mobility may merely be a reflection of an altered starting position.

Addendum: This test may also be performed with the patient supine, but in sitting one can better observe the effect of the weight of the occiput on the joint mechanics.

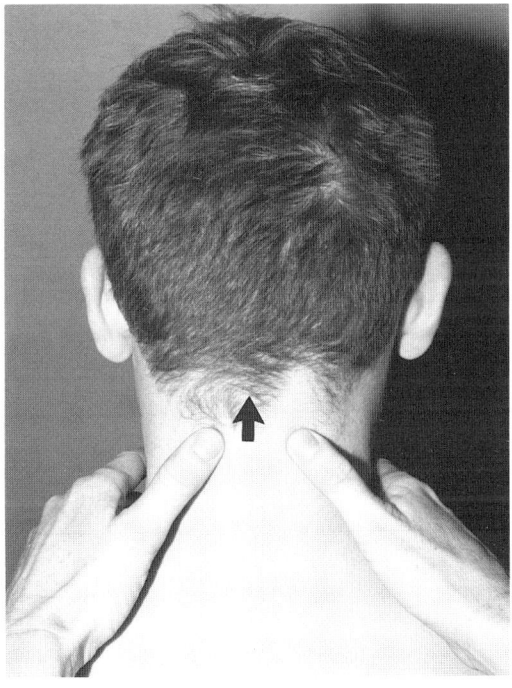

NOTES: _____

_____

_____

_____

_____

ACTIVE MOBILITY TESTS OF OSTEOKINEMATIC FUNCTION

Backward bending

Patient: Sitting.

Therapist: Standing behind the patient.

Palpate: With the thumbs of both hands, palpate the interlaminar spaces of the two adjacent vertebrae.

Test: Instruct the patient to backward bend the head and neck (arrow) and note the quantity of motion as well as the symmetry of motion during extension. When interpreting the mobility findings, the position of the joint at the beginning of the test should be correlated with the subsequent mobility noted since alterations in joint mobility may merely be a reflection of an altered starting position.

Addendum: This test may also be performed with the patient supine, but in sitting one can better observe the effect of the weight of the occiput on the joint mechanics.

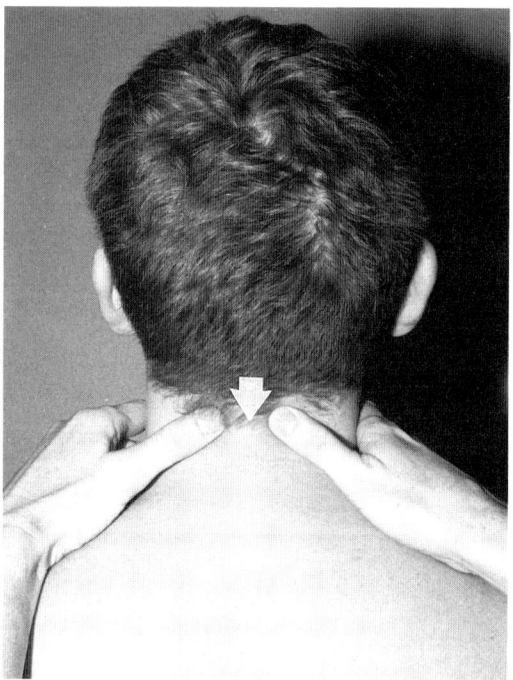

NOTES:

_____

_____

_____

_____

ACTIVE MOBILITY TESTS OF OSTEOKINEMATIC FUNCTION

Lateral bending

Patient: Sitting.

Therapist: Standing behind the patient.

Palpate: With the thumbs of both hands, palpate the interlaminar spaces of the two adjacent vertebrae.

Test: Instruct the patient to laterally bend the head and neck (arrow) and note the quantity and direction of motion. When interpreting the mobility findings, the position of the joint at the beginning of the test should be correlated with the subsequent mobility noted since alterations in joint mobility may merely be a reflection of an altered starting position.

Addendum: This test may also be performed with the patient supine, but in sitting one can better observe the effect of the weight of the occiput on the joint mechanics.

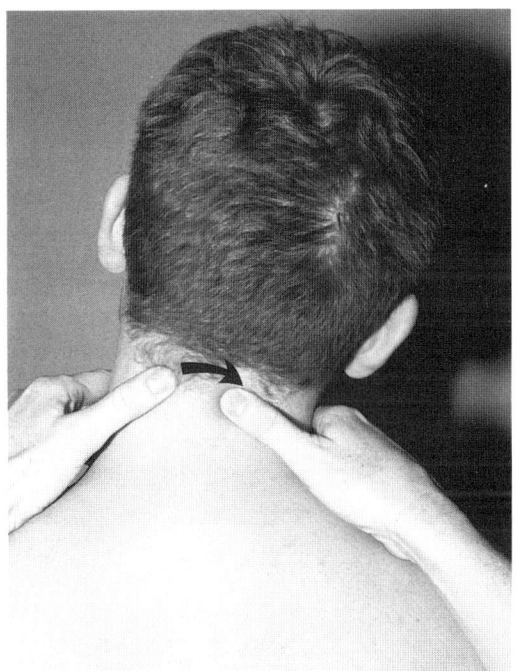

NOTES: _____

_____

_____

_____

_____

ACTIVE MOBILITY TESTS OF OSTEOKINEMATIC FUNCTION

Rotation

Patient: Sitting.

Therapist: Standing behind the patient.

Palpate: With the thumbs of both hands, palpate the interlaminar spaces of the two adjacent vertebrae.

Test: Instruct the patient to rotate the head and neck (arrow) and note the quantity and direction of motion. When interpreting the mobility findings, the position of the joint at the beginning of the test should be correlated with the subsequent mobility noted since alterations in joint mobility may merely be a reflection of an altered starting position.

Addendum: This test may also be performed with the patient supine, but in sitting one can better observe the effect of the weight of the occiput on the joint mechanics.

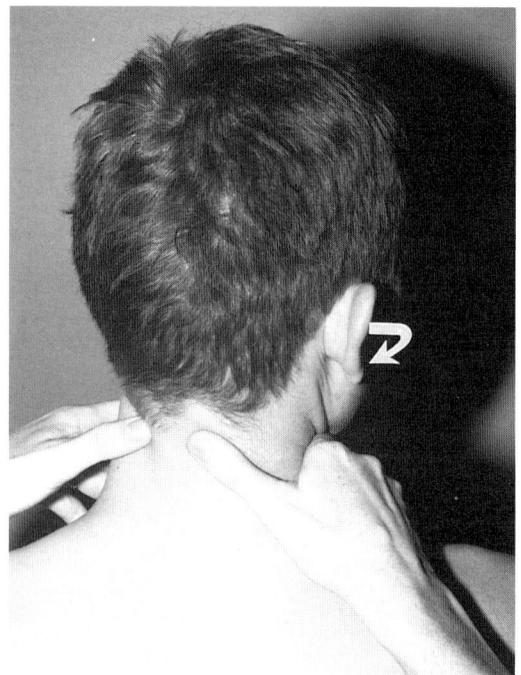

NOTES:

_____

_____

_____

_____

_____

PASSIVE MOBILITY TESTS OF OSTEOKINEMATIC FUNCTION

Flexion/Extension/Lateral bending/Rotation

Patient: Sitting.

Therapist: Standing at the patient's side.

Palpate: With the index and long finger of the dorsal hand, palpate the interlaminar spaces of the segment being assessed. The ulnar border of the fifth finger of the ventral hand is applied to the laminae of the cranial vertebra of the segment being assessed.

Test: Passively flex, extend, laterally bend, rotate the segment and note the quantity, quality, direction of ease and the end feel of motion.

Addendum: This test may also be performed with the patient supine, but in sitting one can better observe the effect of the weight of the occiput on the joint mechanics.

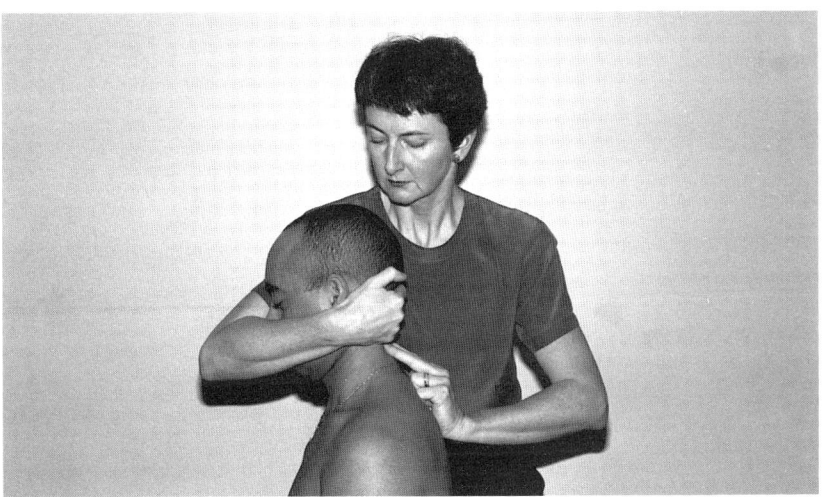

NOTES:

_____

_____

_____

_____

_____

_____

_____

_____

PASSIVE MOBILITY TESTS OF ARTHROKINEMATIC FUNCTION

Lateral translation

Patient:	Sitting.
Therapist:	Standing at the patient's side.
Palpate:	With the thumb and index finger of the dorsal hand, palpate the interlaminar spaces of the segment being assessed. The ulnar border of the fifth finger of the ventral hand is applied to the laminae of the cranial vertebra of the segment being assessed.
Test:	a) Flexion: flex the joint complex and apply a lateral translation force (arrow) to the cranial vertebra. Repeat this test in the opposite direction. Note the quantity, direction of ease and the end feel of motion.
	b) Extension: extend the joint complex and apply a lateral translation force (arrow) to the cranial vertebra. Repeat this test in the opposite direction. Note the quantity, direction of ease and the end feel of motion.
Addendum:	This test may also be performed with the patient supine, but in sitting one can better observe the effect of the weight of the occiput on the joint mechanics.

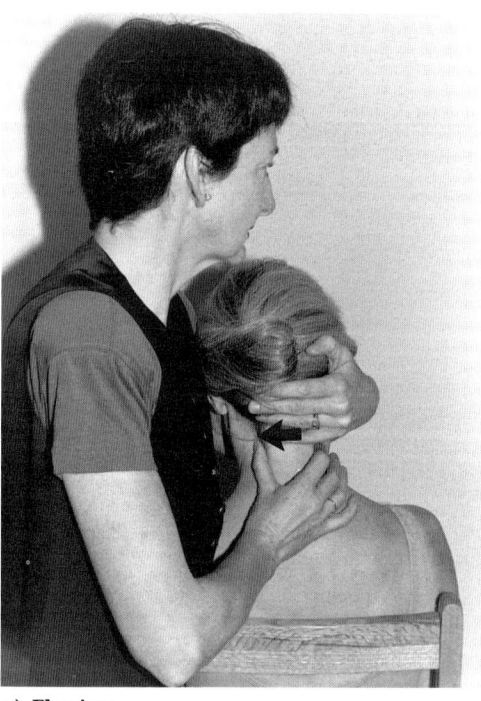

a) Flexion

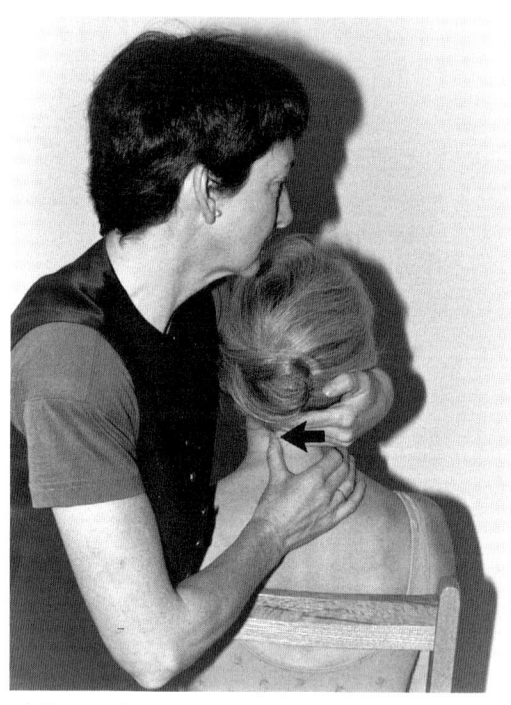

a) Extension

NOTES:

_____

_____

PASSIVE MOBILITY TESTS OF ARTHROKINEMATIC FUNCTION

Superoanterior glide right zygapophysial joint C4-5 – supine

Patient: Supine, head supported on a pillow.
Therapist: Standing at the patient's head facing the shoulders.
Palpate: With a lumbrical grip of the thumb and index finger of the left hand, palpate the articular pillars and laminae of C5. With the right index finger, palpate the right articular pillar of C4.
Test: Fix C5 and apply a force to produce a superoanterior glide (arrow) of the right zygapophysial joint at C4-5 with the right index finger. Note the quantity, direction of ease and the end feel of motion.

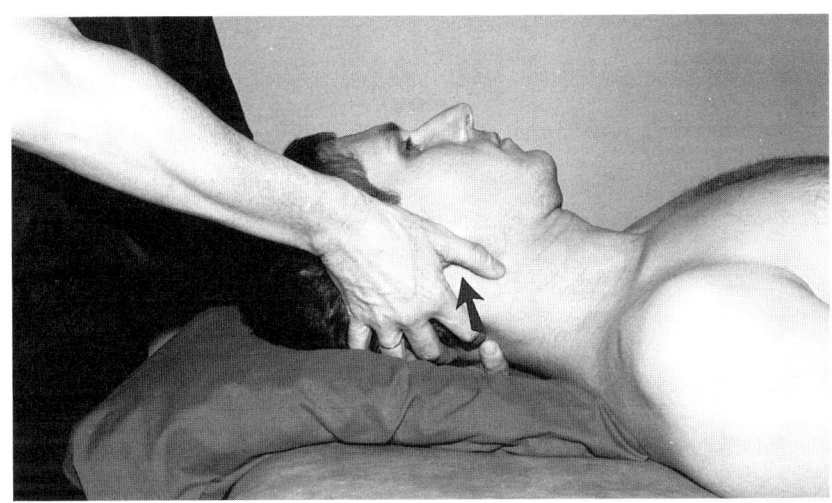

NOTES:
_____
_____
_____
_____
_____
_____
_____
_____
_____
_____

PASSIVE MOBILITY TESTS OF ARTHROKINEMATIC FUNCTION

Superoanterior glide right zygapophysial joint C4-5 – prone

Patient:	Prone, head supported in a neutral position.
Therapist:	Standing beside the patient.
Palpate:	With the thumb and index finger of the left hand, palpate the C5 articular pillars. With the right thumb, palpate the right articular pillar of C4.
Test:	Fix C5 and apply a force to produce a superoanterior glide (arrow) of the right zygapophysial joint at C4-5 with the right thumb. Note the quantity, direction of ease and the end feel of motion.

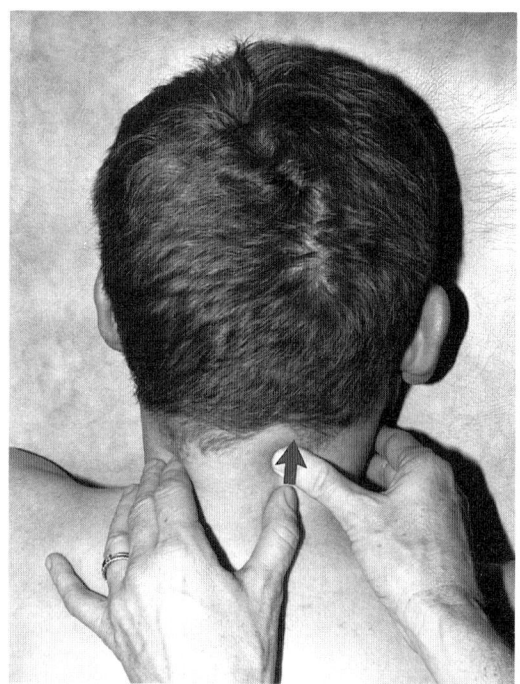

NOTES:

_____

_____

_____

_____

_____

_____

_____

_____

PASSIVE MOBILITY TESTS OF ARTHROKINEMATIC FUNCTION

Superoanteromedial glide right zygapophysial joint C4-5

Patient: Supine, head supported on a pillow.
Therapist: Standing at the patient's head facing the shoulders.
Palpate: With a lumbrical grip of the thumb and index finger of the left hand, palpate the articular pillars and transverse processes of C5. With the right thumb, palpate the anterolateral aspect of the C4 vertebral body on the right. The right index finger palpates the C4 articular pillar on the right.
Test: Fix C5 and apply force to produce a superoanteromedial glide (arrow) of the right zygapophysial joint at C4-5 with the right index finger. Note the quantity, direction of ease and the end feel of motion.

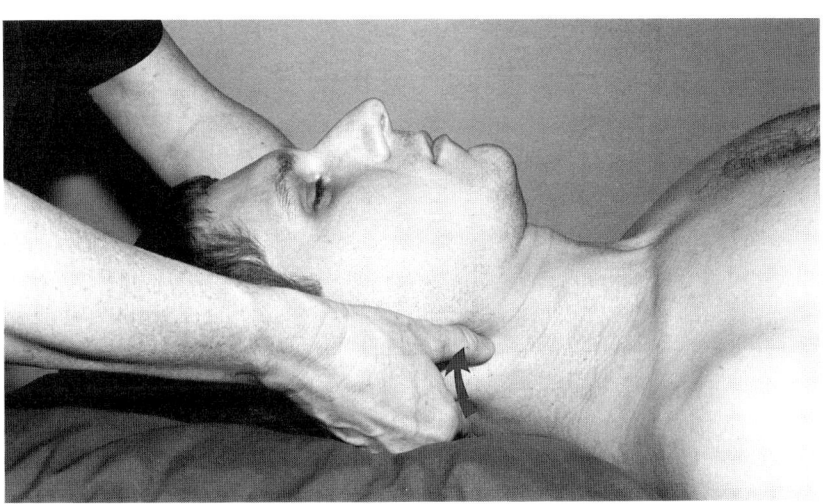

NOTES:

_____

_____

_____

_____

_____

_____

_____

_____

_____

PASSIVE MOBILITY TESTS OF ARTHROKINEMATIC FUNCTION

Inferoposterior glide right zygapophysial joint C4-5

Patient: Supine, head supported on a pillow.

Therapist: Standing at the patient's head facing the shoulders.

Palpate: With a lumbrical grip of the thumb and index finger of the left hand, palpate the articular pillars and laminae of C5. With the right thumb, palpate the anterolateral aspect of the C4 vertebral body on the right. The right index finger palpates the C4 lamina on the right. The rest of this hand supports the cranium and neck cranial to the level being assessed.

Test: Fix C5 and apply a force to produce an inferoposterior glide (arrow) of the right zygapophysial joint at C4-5. Note the quantity, direction of ease and the end feel of motion.

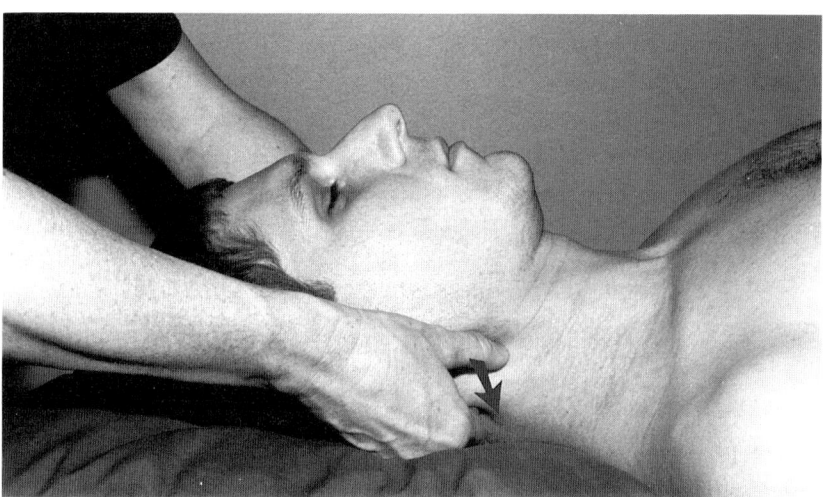

NOTES:

_____

_____

_____

_____

_____

_____

_____

_____

PASSIVE MOBILITY TESTS OF ARTHROKINEMATIC FUNCTION

Inferoposteromedial glide right zygapophysial joint C4-5

Patient: Supine, head supported on a pillow.
Therapist: Standing at the patient's head facing the shoulders.
Palpate: With a lumbrical grip of the thumb and index finger of the left hand, palpate the articular pillars and laminae of the C5 vertebra. With the right thumb, palpate the anterolateral aspect of the C4 vertebral body on the right. The right index finger palpates the C4 lamina on the right.
Test: Fix C5 and apply a force to produce an inferoposteromedial glide (arrow) of the right zygapophysial joint at C4-5. Note the quantity, direction of ease and the end feel of motion.

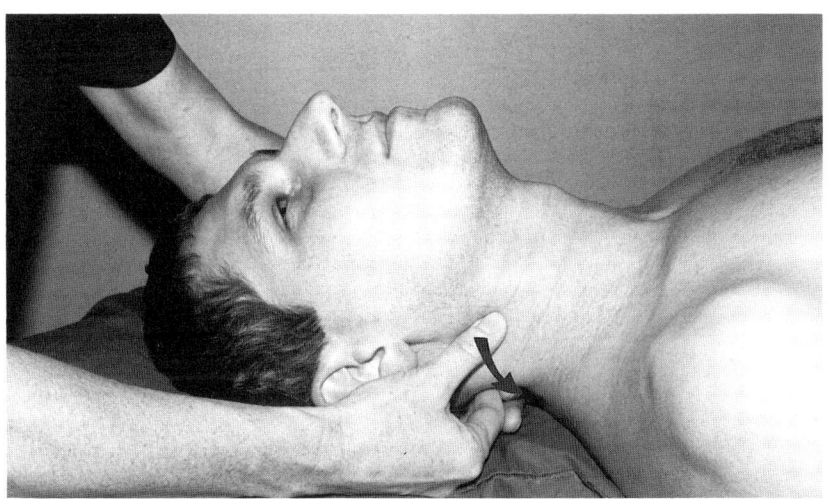

NOTES:

_____

_____

_____

_____

_____

_____

_____

_____

_____

PASSIVE MOBILITY TESTS OF ARTHROKINEMATIC FUNCTION

Anterior glide right uncovertebral joint C4-5

Patient:	Supine, head supported on a pillow.
Therapist:	Standing at the patient's head facing the shoulders.
Palpate:	With the right thumb, palpate the anterolateral aspect of the C4 vertebral body on the right. With the right index finger, palpate the C4 lamina on the right. With the left thumb, palpate the anterolateral aspect of the C5 vertebral body on the left. The left index finger palpates the C5 lamina on the left.
Test:	Fix C5 and apply a force to produce an anterior glide (arrow) of the right uncovertebral joint at C4-5. Note the quantity, direction of ease and the end feel of motion.

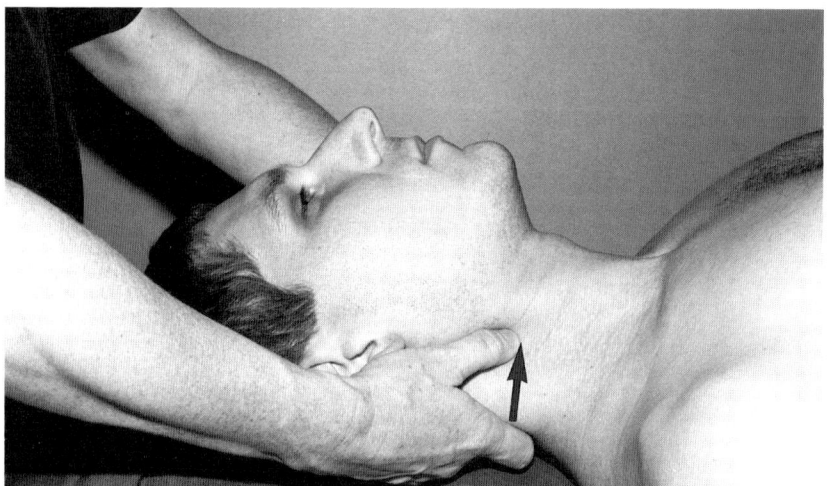

NOTES:

_____

_____

_____

_____

_____

_____

_____

_____

_____

PASSIVE MOBILITY TESTS OF ARTHROKINEMATIC FUNCTION

Posterior glide right uncovertebral joint C4-5

Patient: Supine, head supported on a pillow.

Therapist: Standing at the patient's head facing the shoulders.

Palpate: With the right thumb, palpate the anterolateral aspect of the C4 vertebral body on the right. With the right index finger, palpate the C4 lamina on the right. With the left thumb, palpate the anterolateral aspect of the C5 vertebral body on the left. The left index finger palpates the C5 lamina on the left.

Test: Fix C5 and apply a force to produce a posterior glide (arrow) of the right uncovertebral joint at C4-5. Note the quantity, direction of ease and the end feel of motion.

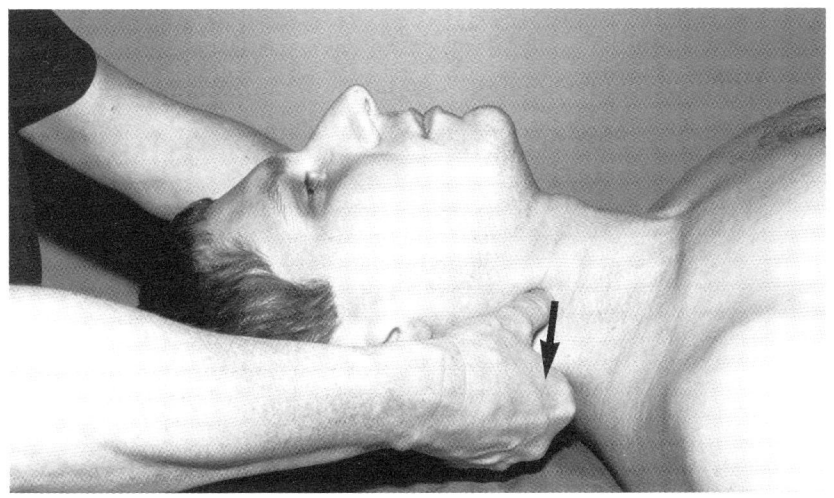

NOTES:

_____

_____

_____

_____

_____

_____

_____

_____

_____

_____

PASSIVE STABILITY TESTS OF ARTHROKINETIC FUNCTION

Vertical (traction/compression) C4-5

Patient: Supine, head supported on a pillow.

Therapist: Standing at the patient's head facing the shoulders.

Palpate: With a lumbrical grip of the index finger and thumb of one hand, palpate the transverse processes, laminae and spinous process of the C5 vertebra. With a lumbrical grip of the index finger and thumb of the other hand, palpate the transverse processes, laminae and spinous process of the C4 vertebra.

Test: Traction: Fix C5 and apply a vertical force (arrow) in a cranial direction to the C4 vertebra. Note the reproduction of any symptoms. Repeat the test in varying degrees of flexion and extension of the C4-5 joint complex.

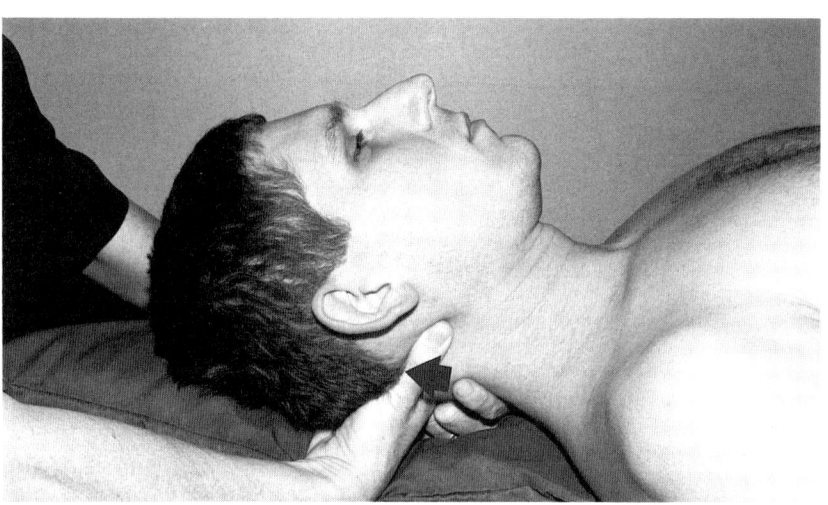

Traction

Continued on Page 87

NOTES:

_____

_____

_____

_____

_____

_____

_____

_____

MIDCERVICAL REGION

Compression: Traction C5 vertically and note the reproduction of any symptoms. Apply a vertical compression force (arrow) in a caudal direction to the C4-5 joint complex. Note the reproduction of any symptoms. Repeat the test in varying degrees of flexion and extension of the C4-5 joint complex.

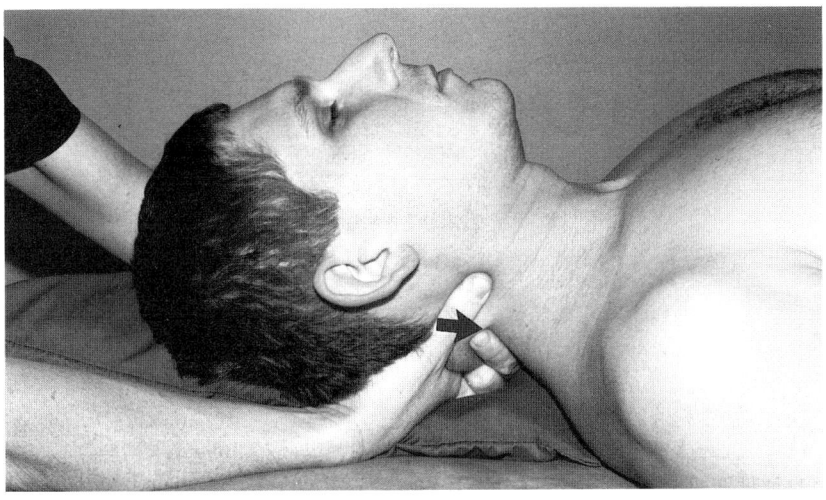

Compression

NOTES:

_____

_____

_____

_____

_____

_____

_____

_____

_____

_____

_____

_____

_____

_____

_____

PASSIVE STABILITY TESTS OF ARTHROKINETIC FUNCTION

Anterior translation C4-5

Patient:	Supine, head supported on a pillow.
Therapist:	Standing at the patient's head facing the shoulders.
Palpate:	With the thumbs, palpate the anterior aspect of the transverse processes of C5. With the radial border of the index fingers, palpate the laminae and spinous process of the C4 vertebra.
Test:	Fix C5 with the thumbs and apply a posteroanterior force (arrow) to the C4 vertebra to produce an anterior translation at C4-5 in a PURE horizontal plane. Sustain the force until the end feel is perceived. Note the quantity and the end feel of motion as well as the reproduction of any symptoms.

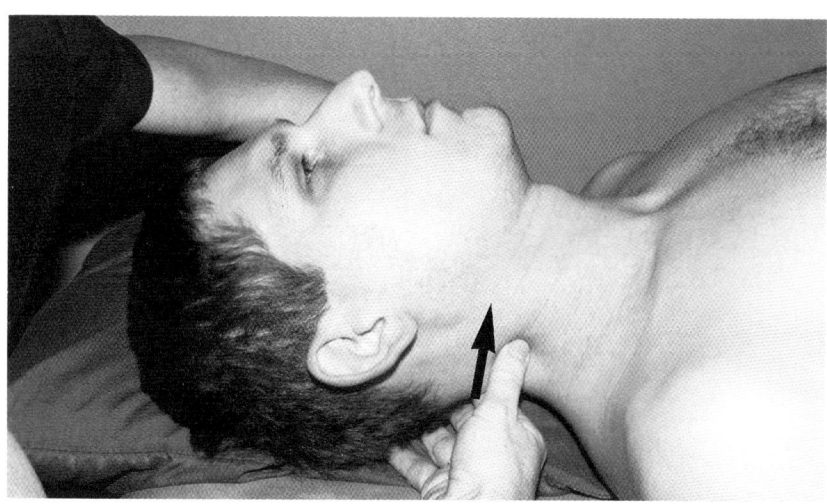

NOTES:

_____

_____

_____

_____

_____

_____

_____

_____

_____

PASSIVE STABILITY TESTS OF ARTHROKINETIC FUNCTION

Posterior translation C4-5

Patient:	Supine, head supported on a pillow.
Therapist:	Standing at the patient's head facing the shoulders.
Palpate:	With the radial border of both index fingers, palpate the spinous process and laminae of the C5 vertebra. With the thumbs, palpate the anterior aspect of the transverse processes of the C4 vertebra.
Test:	Fix C5 and apply an anteroposterior force (arrow) to the C4 transverse processes to produce a posterior translation of C4-5 in a PURE horizontal plane. Sustain the force until the end feel is perceived. Note the quantity and the end feel of motion as well as the reproduction of any symptoms.

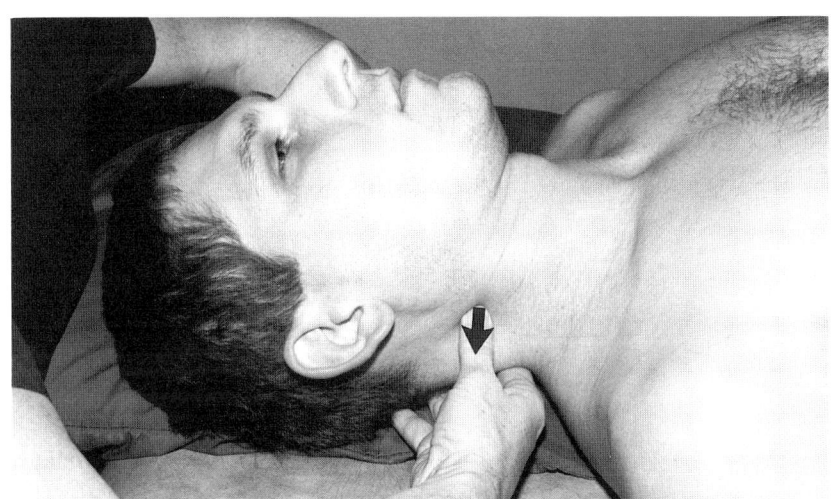

NOTES:

_____

_____

_____

_____

_____

_____

_____

_____

_____

_____

PASSIVE STABILITY TESTS OF ARTHROKINETIC FUNCTION

Right lateral translation C4-5

Patient:	Supine, head supported on a pillow.
Therapist:	Standing at the patient's head facing the shoulders.
Palpate:	With the radial border of the MCP joint of the right index finger, palpate the right transverse process of the C5 vertebra. With the radial border of the MCP joint of the left index finger, palpate the left transverse process of the C4 vertebra.
Test:	Fix C5 and apply a right lateral translation force (arrow) to the C4 vertebra in a PURE horizontal plane with the left index finger. Sustain the force until the end feel is perceived. Note the quantity and the end feel of motion as well as the reproduction of any symptoms.

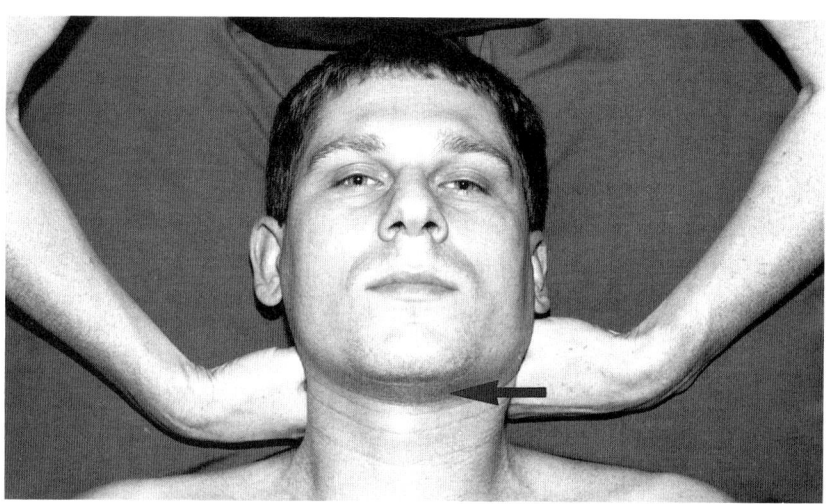

NOTES:

_____

_____

_____

_____

_____

_____

_____

_____

_____

_____

PASSIVE STABILITY TESTS OF ARTHROKINETIC FUNCTION

Right torsion C4-5

Patient:	Supine, head supported on a pillow.
Therapist:	Standing at the patient's head facing the shoulders.
Palpate:	With the left thumb, palpate the anterior aspect of the left transverse process of the C5 vertebra. With the right thumb, palpate the anterior aspect of the right transverse process of the C4 vertebra.
Test:	Fix C5 and apply an anteroposterior force (arrow) to the right transverse process of C4, to produce right torsion at C4-5. Sustain the force until the end feel is perceived. Note the quantity and the end feel of motion as well as the reproduction of any symptoms.

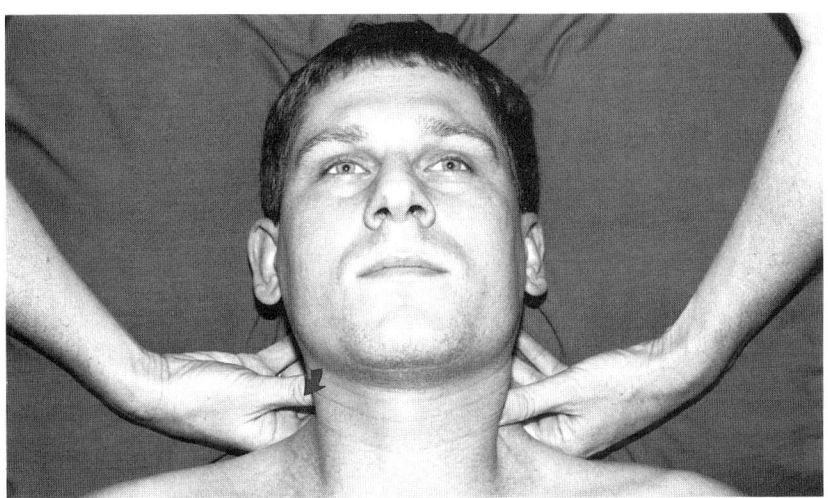

NOTES:

_____

_____

_____

_____

_____

_____

_____

_____

_____

MOBILIZATION TECHNIQUES

Restriction of flexion (superoanterior glide) C4-5

Patient: Sitting.

Therapist: Standing beside the patient.

Palpate: With a lumbrical grip of the index finger and thumb of the dorsal hand, palpate the transverse processes and laminae of the C5 vertebra. The rest of the hand supports the lower cervical spine. The ulnar border of the fifth finger of the ventral hand is applied to the laminae and inferior articular processes of the C4 vertebra. The rest of the hand supports the cranium and the upper cervical spine.

Localization: Fix C5 with the dorsal hand and flex C4-5 to the motion barrier.

Mobilization: **Passive** – Apply a grade 1 to 4 force to the C4 vertebra to produce a superoanterior glide (arrow) at the zygapophyseal joints thus flexing the C4-5 joint complex.
Active – From the motion barrier, instruct the patient to turn the eyes in a direction which facilitates further flexion at C4-5. The isometric contraction is held for up to 5 seconds and followed by a period of complete relaxation. The joint is then passively taken to the new motion barrier. This technique is repeated 3 times and followed by a re-evaluation of osteokinematic, arthrokinematic and arthrokinetic function.

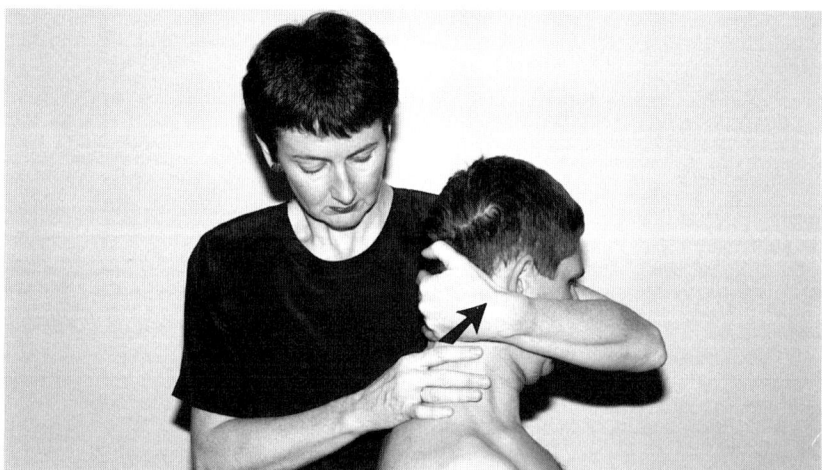

NOTES: _____

_____

_____

MOBILIZATION TECHNIQUES

Restriction of flexion/left lateral bending/rotation (superoanteromedial glide right zygapophysial joint) C4-5 – supine

Ipsilateral technique

Patient: Supine, head supported on a pillow.

Therapist: Standing at the patient's head facing the shoulders.

Palpate: With the radial aspect of the right index finger, palpate the inferior articular process and lamina of the C4 vertebra on the right. With the other hand, support the cranium and neck cranial to the level being treated.

Localization: An incongruent lock of the cranial segment is accomplished by right lateral bending and left rotating the C3-4 joint complex, leaving the craniovertebral joints in a neutral position. The motion barrier for flexion, left rotation, left lateral bending of C4-5 is localized by passively gliding the right inferior articular process of the C4 vertebra superoanteromedially on the superior articular process of C5.

Continued on Page 94

NOTES:

_____

_____

_____

_____

_____

_____

_____

_____

_____

_____

_____

_____

_____

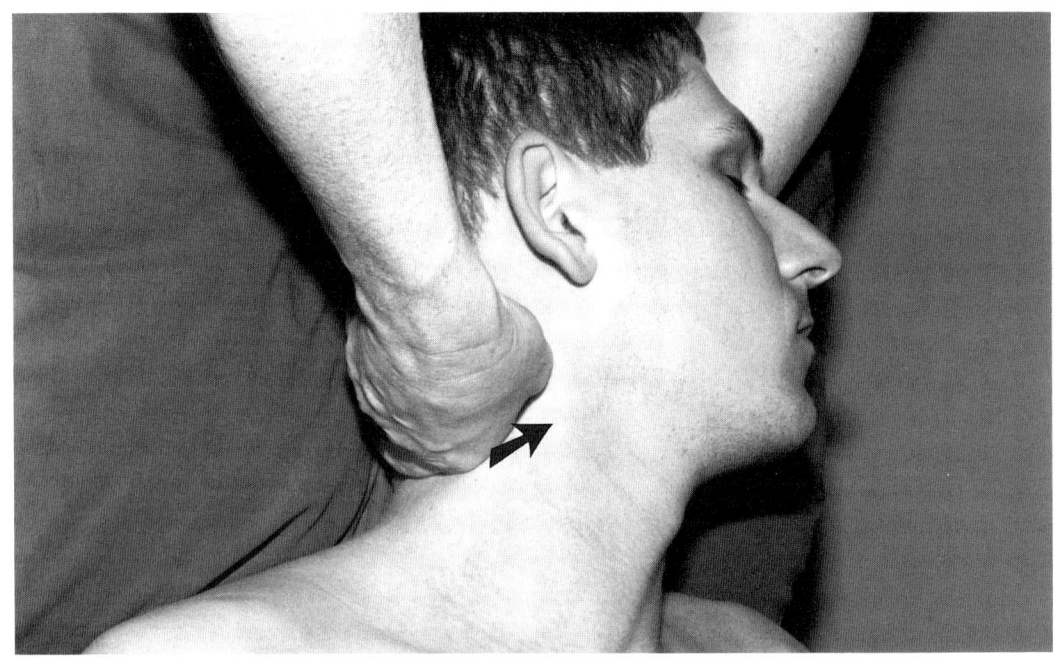

Mobilization: **Passive** – Apply a grade 1 to 5 force to the C4 vertebra to produce a superoanteromedial glide (arrow) of the right zygapophysial joint at C4-5.

Active – From the motion barrier, instruct the patient to turn the eyes in a direction which facilitates further flexion/left lateral bending/rotation at C4-5. The isometric contraction is held for up to 5 seconds and followed by a period of complete relaxation. The joint is then passively taken to the new motion barrier. This technique is repeated 3 times and followed by a re-evaluation of osteokinematic, arthrokinematic and arthrokinetic function.

Addendum: This technique is inappropriate in the presence of hypermobility either proximal or distal to the joint being mobilized.

NOTES:

_____

_____

_____

_____

_____

_____

_____

MOBILIZATION TECHNIQUES

Restriction of flexion/left lateral bending/rotation (superoanteromedial glide right zygapophysial joint) C4-5 – supine

Contralateral technique

Patient: Supine, head supported on a pillow.

Therapist: Standing at the patient's head facing the shoulders.

Palpate: With the radial aspect of the left index finger, palpate the inferior articular process and lamina of the C4 vertebra on the left. With the other hand, support the cranium and neck cranial to the level being treated.

Localization: An incongruent lock of the cranial segment is accomplished by left lateral bending and right rotating the C3-4 joint complex, leaving the craniovertebral joints in a neutral position. Flex C4-5 to the motion barrier. Full superoanteromedial glide of the right zygapophysial joint is achieved by left rotating and left lateral bending the C4 on C5 vertebra from this position of full flexion.

Mobilization: Passive – A grade 1 to 5 force is applied to C4 with the left index finger to produce an inferoposteromedial glide (arrow) of the left zygapophysial joint at C4-5 and, therefore, a superoanteromedial glide of the right zygapophysial joint at C4-5.

Active – From the motion barrier, instruct the patient to turn the eyes in a direction which facilitates further flexion/left lateral bending/rotation at C4-5. The isometric contraction is held for up to 5 seconds and followed by a period of complete relaxation. The joint is then passively taken to the new motion barrier. This technique is repeated 3 times and followed by a re-evaluation of osteokinematic, arthrokinematic, and arthrokinetic function.

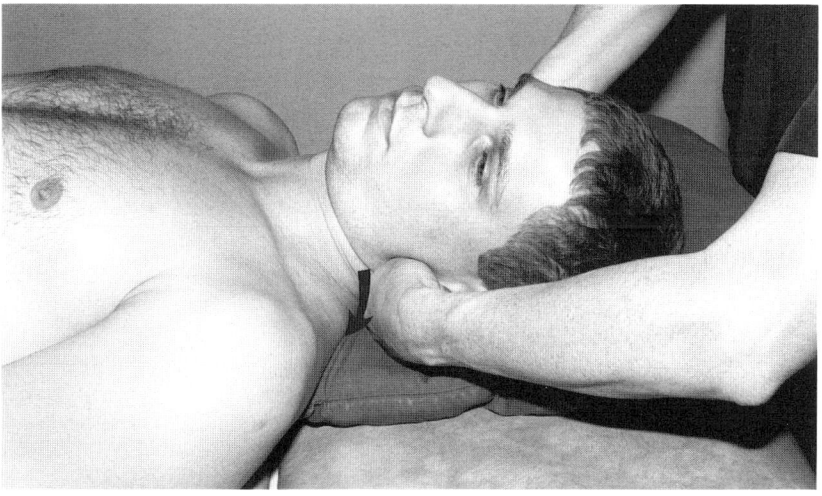

MOBILIZATION TECHNIQUES

Restriction of flexion/left lateral bending/rotation (superoanteromedial glide right zygapophysial joint) C4-5 – sitting

Patient:	Sitting.
Therapist:	Standing beside the patient.
Palpate:	With a lumbrical grip of the thumb and index finger of the dorsal hand, palpate the spinous process and the laminae of the C5 vertebra. With the ulnar border of the fifth finger of the ventral hand, palpate the inferior articular process of the C4 vertebra on the right.
Localization:	Fix C5. An incongruent lock of the cranial segment is accomplished by right lateral bending and left rotating the C3-4 joint complex, leaving the craniovertebral joints in a neutral position. This position is maintained by support from the forearm of the ventral hand. Flex, left lateral bend, left rotate the C4-5 joint complex to the motion barrier.
Mobilization:	**Passive** – Apply a grade 1 to 4 force to the C4 vertebra to produce a superoanteromedial glide (arrow) of the right zygapophysial joint at C4-5. **Active** – From the motion barrier, instruct the patient to turn the eyes in a direction which facilitates further flexion/left lateral bending/rotation at C4-5. The isometric contraction is held for up to 5 seconds and followed by a period of complete relaxation. The joint is then passively taken to the new motion barrier. This technique is repeated 3 times and followed by a re-evaluation of osteokinematic, arthrokinematic, and arthrokinetic function.

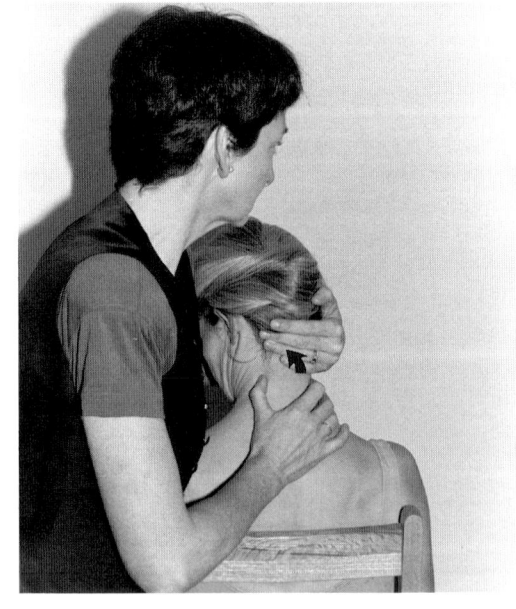

MOBILIZATION TECHNIQUES

Restriction of extension (posteroinferior glide) C4-5

Patient:	Sitting.
Therapist:	Standing beside the patient.
Palpate:	With a lumbrical grip of the index finger and thumb, palpate the transverse processes and laminae of the C5 vertebra. The rest of the hand supports the lower cervical spine. The ulnar border of the fifth finger of the ventral hand is applied to the laminae and inferior articular processes of the C4 vertebra. The rest of the hand supports the cranium and the upper cervical spine.
Localization:	Fix C5 and extend the C4-5 joint complex to the motion barrier.
Mobilization:	**Passive** – Apply a grade 1 to 4 force to the C4 vertebra to produce a posteroinferior glide (arrow) of the zygapophyseal joints at C4-5.
	Active – From the motion barrier, instruct the patient to turn the eyes in a direction which facilitates further extension at C4-5. The isometric contraction is held for up to 5 seconds and followed by a period of complete relaxation. The joint is then passively taken to the new motion barrier. This technique is repeated 3 times and followed by a re-evaluation of osteokinematic, arthrokinematic, and arthrokinetic function.

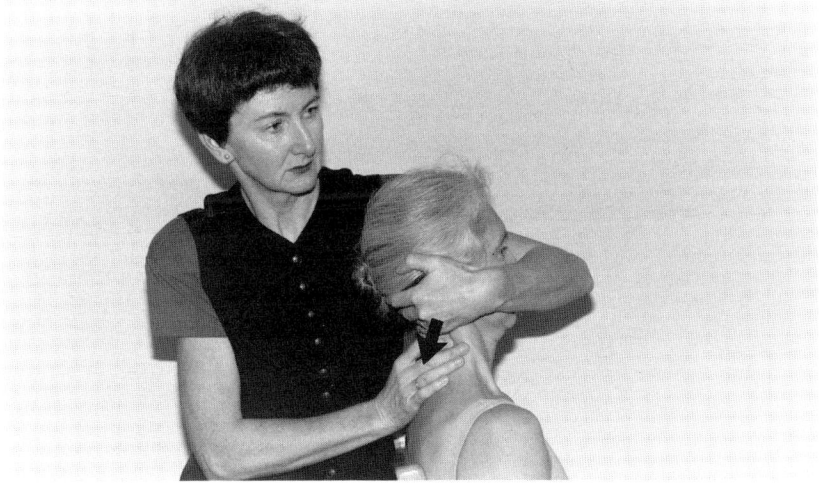

NOTES:

_____

_____

_____

MOBILIZATION TECHNIQUES

Restriction of extension/right lateral bending/rotation (posteroinferomedial glide right zygapophysial joint) C4-5 – supine

Patient:	Supine, head supported on a pillow.
Therapist:	Standing at the patient's head facing the shoulders.
Palpate:	With the radial aspect of the right index finger, palpate the spinous process and the right inferior articular process of the C4 vertebra. With the other hand, support the cranium and neck cranial to the level being treated.
Localization:	An incongruent lock of the cranial segment is accomplished by right lateral bending and left rotating the C3-4 joint complex, leaving the craniovertebral joints in a neutral position. The motion barrier for extension/right lateral bending/right rotation of C4-5 is then localized by pushing the right inferior articular process of C4 posteroinferomedially on C5.
Mobilization:	**Passive** – Apply a grade 1 to 5 force to the C4 vertebra to produce a posteroinferomedial glide (arrow) of the right zygapophysial joint at C4-5.
	Active – From the motion barrier, instruct the patient to turn the eyes in a direction which facilitates further extension/right lateral bending/right rotation. The isometric contraction is held for up to 5 seconds and followed by a period of complete relaxation. The joint is then passively taken to the new motion barrier. This technique is repeated 3 times and followed by a re-evaluation of osteokinematic, arthrokinematic, and arthrokinetic function.

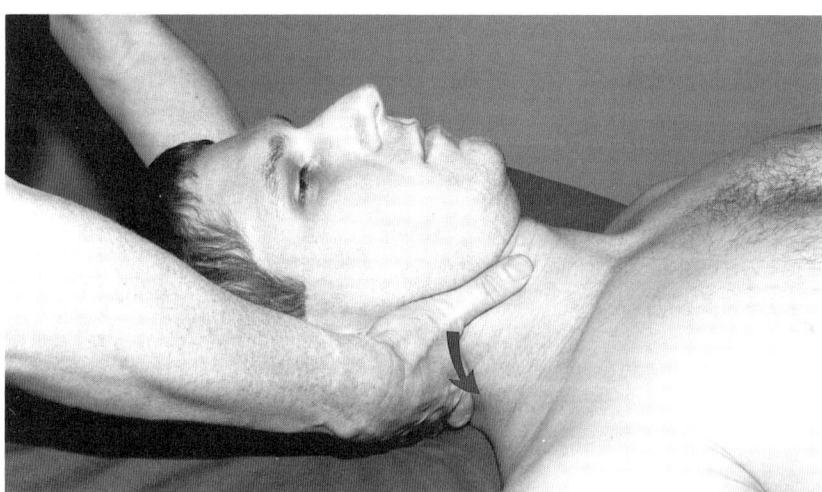

NOTES:

_____

_____

MOBILIZATION TECHNIQUES

Restriction of extension/right lateral bending/rotation (posteroinferomedial glide right zygapophysial joint) C4-5 – sitting

Patient: Sitting.

Therapist: Standing at the patient's side.

Palpate: With a lumbrical grip of the thumb and the index finger of the dorsal hand, palpate the spinous process and laminae of the C5 vertebra. The ulnar border of the fifth finger of the ventral hand is applied to the right lamina and inferior articular process of the C4 vertebra.

Localization: An incongruent lock of the cranial segment is accomplished by right lateral bending and left rotating the C3-4 joint complex leaving the craniovertebral joints in a neutral position. From this position, the motion barrier is localized by passively pushing the right inferior articular process of C4 posteroinferomedially on C5.

Mobilization: **Passive** – Apply a grade 1 to 4 force to the C4 vertebra to produce a posteroinferomedial glide (arrow) of the right zygapophysial joint at C4-5.

Active – From the motion barrier, instruct the patient to turn the eyes in a direction which facilitates further extension/right lateral bending/right rotation at C4-5. The isometric contraction is held for up to 5 seconds and followed by a period of complete relaxation. The joint is then passively taken to the new motion barrier. This technique is repeated 3 times and followed by a re-evaluation of osteokinematic, arthrokinematic and arthrokinetic function.

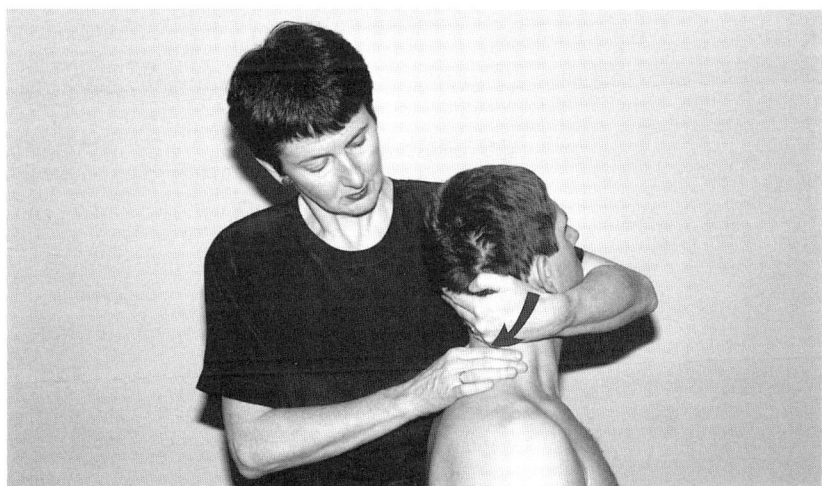

NOTES:

_____

_____

MOBILIZATION TECHNIQUES

Restriction of flexion (anterior glide) right C4-5 uncovertebral joint

Patient: Supine, head supported on a pillow.

Therapist: Standing at the patient's head facing the shoulders.

Palpate: With the right thumb, palpate the anterolateral aspect of the C4 vertebral body on the right. With the right index finger, palpate the C4 lamina on the right. With the left thumb, palpate the anterolateral aspect of the C5 vertebral body on the left. The left index finger palpates the C5 lamina on the left.

Localization: Flex the C4-5 joint complex to the motion barrier and fix the C5 vertebra on the left.

Mobilization: **Passive** – Apply a grade 1 to 5 posteroanterior force (arrow) to the right C4 vertebra, thus producing an anterior glide of the right uncovertebral joint.

    Active – From the motion barrier, instruct the patient to turn the eyes in a direction which facilitates further flexion of the right uncovertebral joint. The isometric contraction is held for up to 5 seconds and followed by a period of complete relaxation. The joint is then passively taken to the new motion barrier. This technique is repeated 3 times and followed by a re-evaluation of osteokinematic, arthrokinematic and arthrokinetic function.

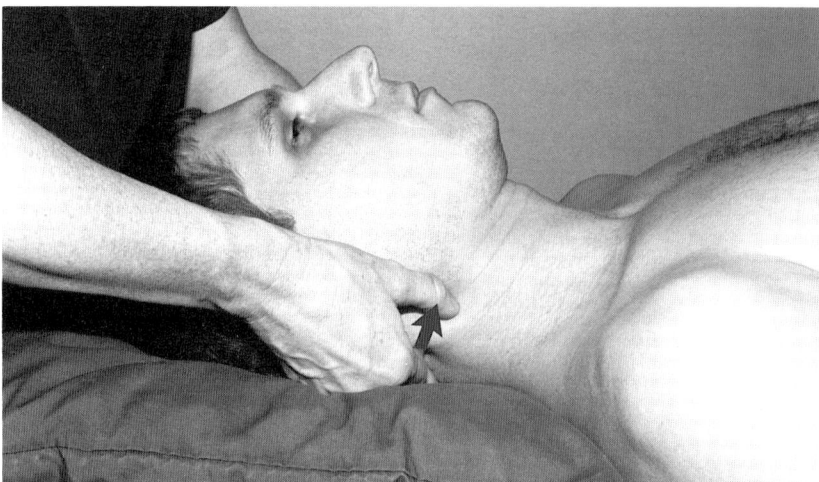

NOTES:

_____

_____

_____

MOBILIZATION TECHNIQUES

Restriction of extension (posterior glide) right C4-5 uncovertebral joint

Patient:	Supine, head supported on a pillow.
Therapist:	Standing at the patient's head facing the shoulders.
Palpate:	With the right thumb, palpate the anterolateral aspect of the C4 vertebral body on the right. With the right index finger, palpate the C4 lamina on the right. With the left thumb, palpate the anterolateral aspect of the C5 vertebral body on the left. The left index finger palpates the C5 lamina on the left.
Localization:	Flex the C4-5 joint complex to the motion barrier and fix the C5 vertebra on the left.
Mobilization:	**Passive** – Apply a grade 1 to 5 anteroposterior force (arrow) to the right C4 vertebra, thus producing an posterior glide of the right uncovertebral joint at C4-5.
	Active – From the motion barrier, instruct the patient to turn the eyes in a direction which facilitates further extension of the right C4-5 uncovertebral joint. The isometric contraction is held for up to 5 seconds and followed by a period of complete relaxation. The joint is then passively taken to the new motion barrier. This technique is repeated 3 times and followed by a re-evaluation of osteokinematic, arthrokinematic and arthrokinetic function.

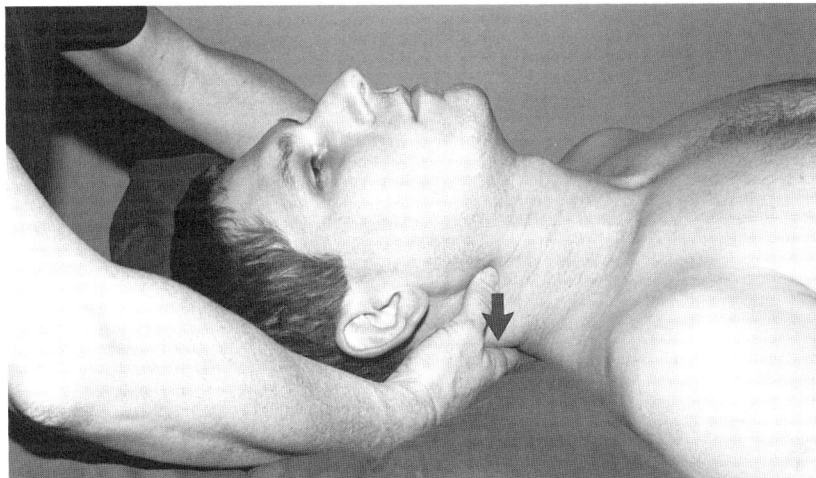

NOTES:

_____

_____

_____

MOBILIZATION TECHNIQUES

Right lateral shift lesion C4-5

Patient: Supine, head supported on a pillow.

Therapist: Standing at the patient's head facing the shoulders.

Palpate: With the radial aspect of the index finger, palpate the transverse process and the lamina of the C4 vertebra on the right. With the other hand, support the cranium and neck above the level being treated.

Localization: An incongruent lock of the cranial segment is accomplished by right lateral bending and left rotating the C3-4 joint complex leaving the craniovertebral joints in a neutral position. Then, apply a longitudinal traction force to the C4-5 joint complex. Maintain the traction and localize the motion barrier by passively gliding C4 on C5 to the left in a medioinferior direction (in the plane of the uncovertebral joint) using the right index finger.

Mobilization: From the motion barrier, a grade 4 to 5 force is applied to the right lateral aspect of the C4 vertebra in a medial and inferior direction (arrow), thus producing left lateral translation at C4-5.

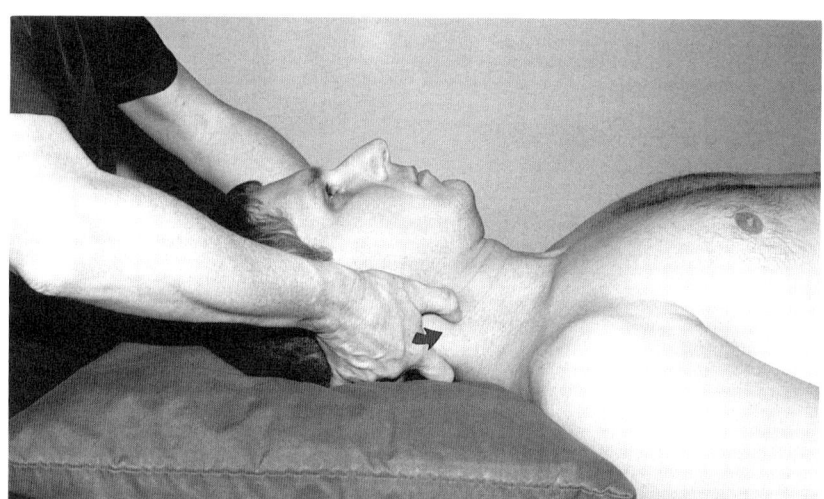

NOTES:

_____

_____

_____

_____

_____

MOBILIZATION TECHNIQUES

Regional traction

Patient: Supine, head supported on a pillow.

Therapist: Standing at the patient's head facing the shoulders.

Palpate: With one hand, support the occiput and craniovertebral joints. With the other hand, cradle the mandible. If a TMJ dysfunction exists, cradle the occiput with both hands.

Localization: The degree of cervical flexion determines the level of localization.

Mobilization: Apply a grade 1 to 4 traction force by slowly leaning backwards. The hand supporting the mandible is used only to guide the movement thus avoiding compression of the temporomandibular joints.

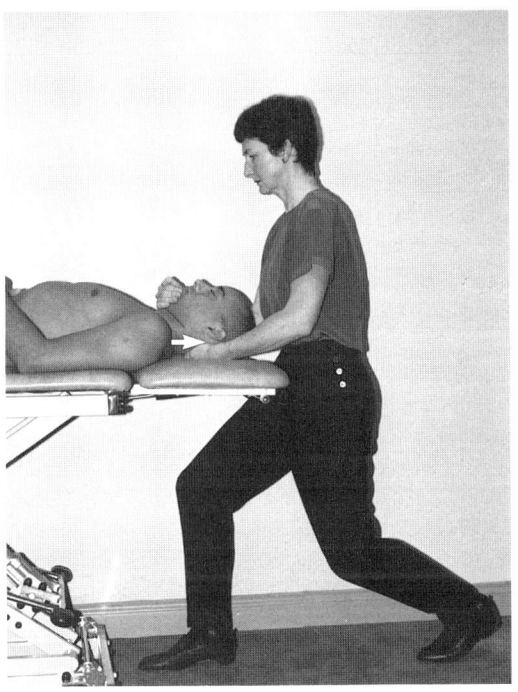

NOTES:

_____

_____

_____

_____

_____

_____

MOBILIZATION TECHNIQUES

Specific traction C4-5

Patient:	Sitting.
Therapist:	Standing at the patient's side, hips and knees flexed.
Palpate:	With a lumbrical grip of the index finger and thumb of the dorsal hand, palpate the laminae and transverse processes of C5. The rest of this hand supports the lower cervical spine. The ulnar border of the fifth finger of the ventral hand is applied to the laminae and inferior articular processes of C4. The rest of this hand supports the cranium and the upper cervical spine.
Localization:	An incongruent lock of the cranial segment is accomplished by right lateral bending and left rotating the C3-4 joint complex, leaving the craniovertebral joints in a neutral position.
Mobilization:	Fix C5 and apply a vertical traction force (arrow) to the C4-5 joint complex.

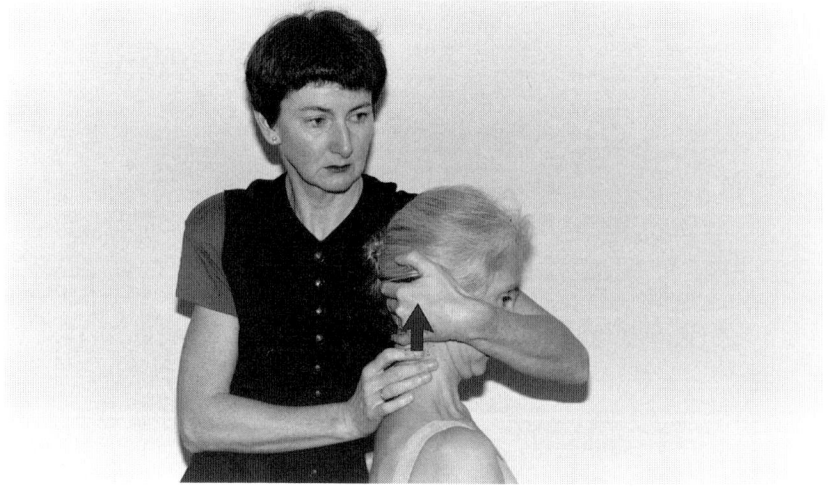

NOTES:

_____

_____

_____

_____

_____

_____

_____

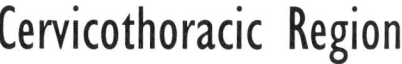
Cervicothoracic Region

CERVICOTHORACIC REGION

ASSESSMENT

POSITIONAL TESTS — SPINAL

Patient: Sitting.
Therapist: Standing behind the patient.
Palpate: With the thumbs, palpate the transverse processes of the T1 vertebra.
Test: a) Flex the joint complex and assess the position of the T1 vertebra relative to T2 by noting which transverse process is the most dorsal. A dorsal left transverse process of T1 relative to T2 is indicative of a left rotated position of the T1-2 joint complex in flexion.
b) Extend the joint complex and assess the position of the T1 vertebra relative to T2 by noting which transverse process is the most dorsal. A dorsal left transverse process of T1 relative to T2 is indicative of a left rotated position of the T1-2 joint complex in extension.

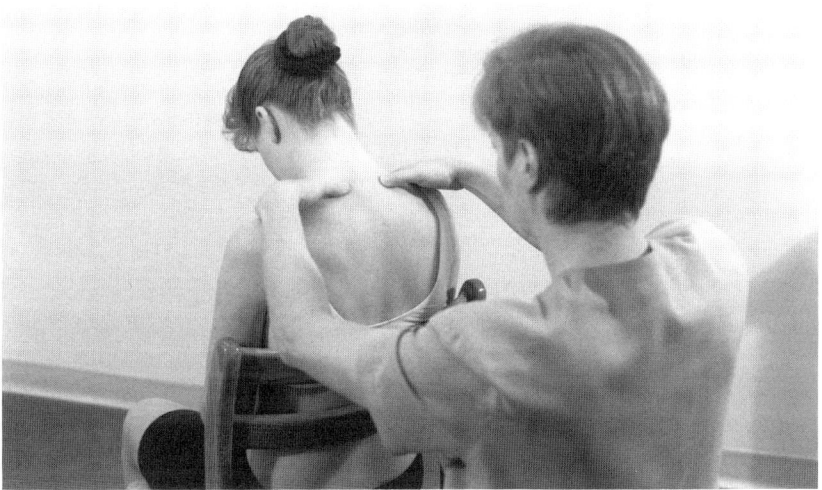

NOTES:

_____
_____
_____
_____
_____
_____
_____
_____
_____

POSITIONAL TESTS – COSTAL

Patient: Sitting.

Dorsal
Therapist: Standing behind the patient.
Palpate: With the thumbs, palpate the ribs just lateral to the tubercle and medial to the angle.

Ventral
Therapist: Standing in front of the patient.
Palpate: **First rib** – With the index fingers or thumbs, palpate the ventral aspect of the first ribs at the manubriocostal junction.
Second rib – With the index fingers or thumbs, palpate the ventral and then the cranial aspect of the second ribs at the manubriocostal junction.
Test: Note the craniocaudal, ventrodorsal relationship of the two ribs, left and right.

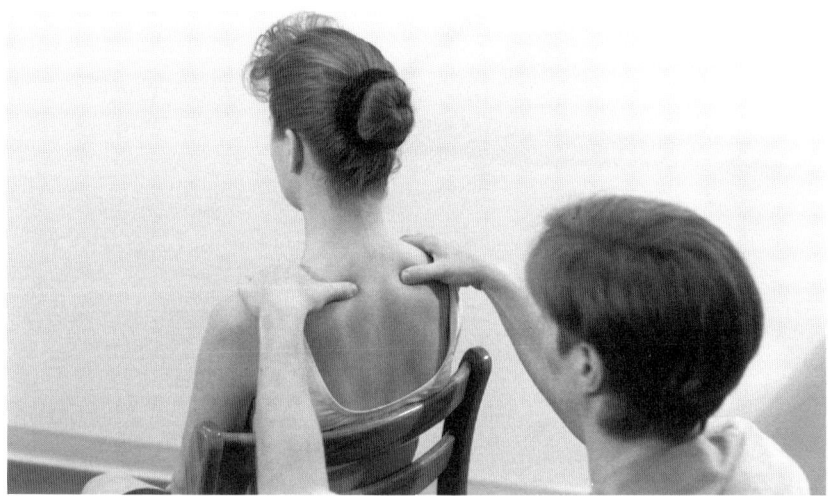

NOTES:

_____
_____
_____
_____
_____
_____
_____
_____
_____

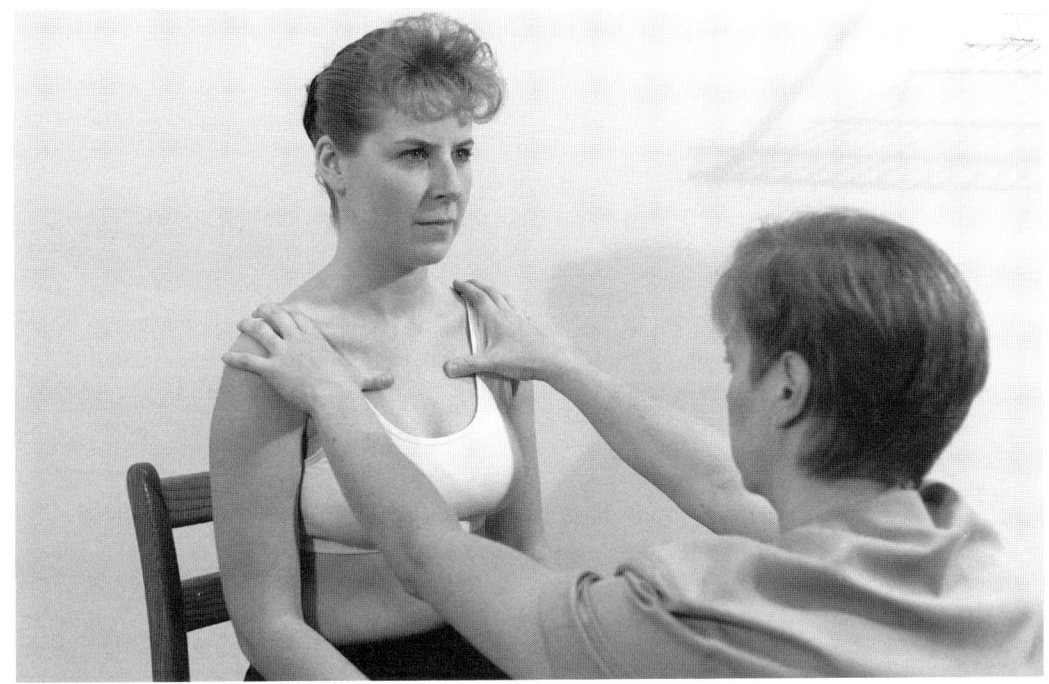

NOTES:

_____

_____

_____

_____

_____

_____

_____

_____

_____

_____

_____

_____

_____

_____

_____

_____

_____

ACTIVE MOBILITY TESTS OF OSTEOKINEMATIC FUNCTION — SPINAL

Forward bending

Patient: Sitting.

Therapist: Standing behind the patient.

Palpate: With the index finger and thumb of both hands, palpate the transverse processes of two adjacent vertebrae.

Test: Instruct the patient to forward bend the head and neck and note the quantity of motion as well as the symmetry of motion during flexion. Both index fingers should travel superiorly an equal distance. When interpreting the mobility findings, the position of the joint at the beginning of the test should be correlated with the subsequent mobility noted since alterations in joint mobility may merely be a reflection of an altered starting position.

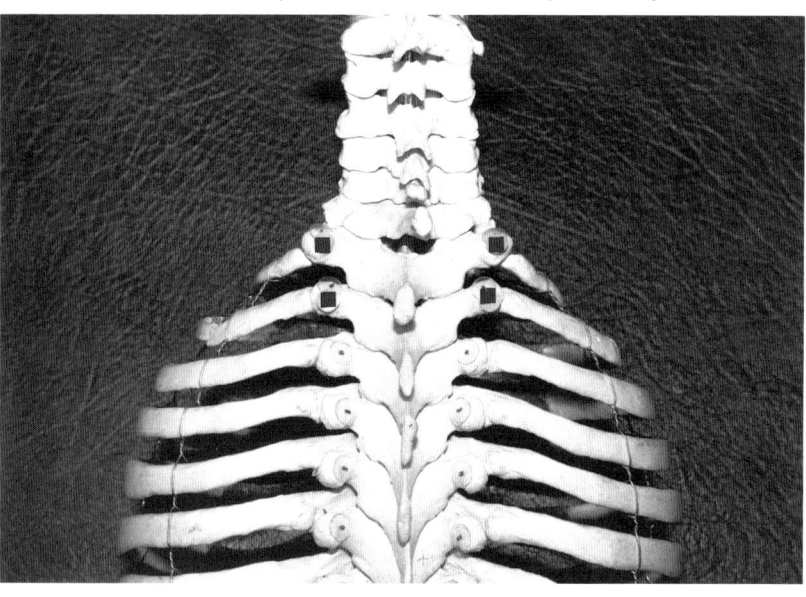
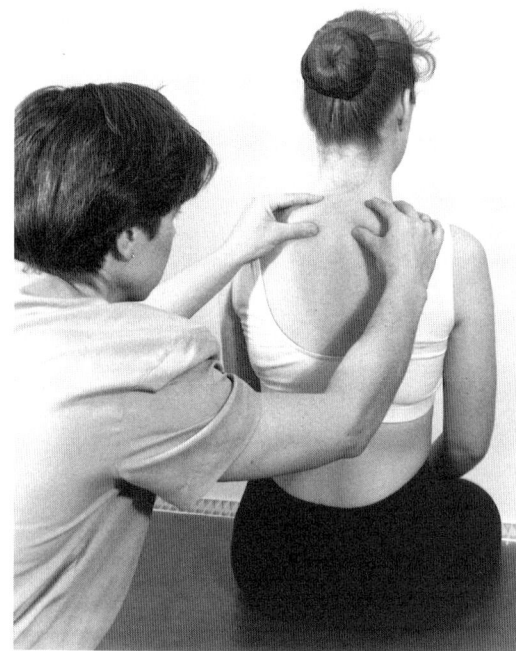

NOTES:

_____

_____

_____

_____

_____

_____

ACTIVE MOBILITY TESTS OF OSTEOKINEMATIC FUNCTION — SPINAL

Backward bending

Patient:	Sitting.
Therapist:	Standing behind the patient.
Palpate:	With the index finger and thumb of both hands, palpate the transverse processes of two adjacent vertebrae.
Test:	Instruct the patient to elevate both arms and note the quantity of motion as well as the symmetry of motion during extension. Both index fingers should travel posteroinferiorly an equal distance. When interpreting the mobility findings, the position of the joint at the beginning of the test should be correlated with the subsequent mobility noted since alterations in joint mobility may merely be a reflection of an altered starting position.

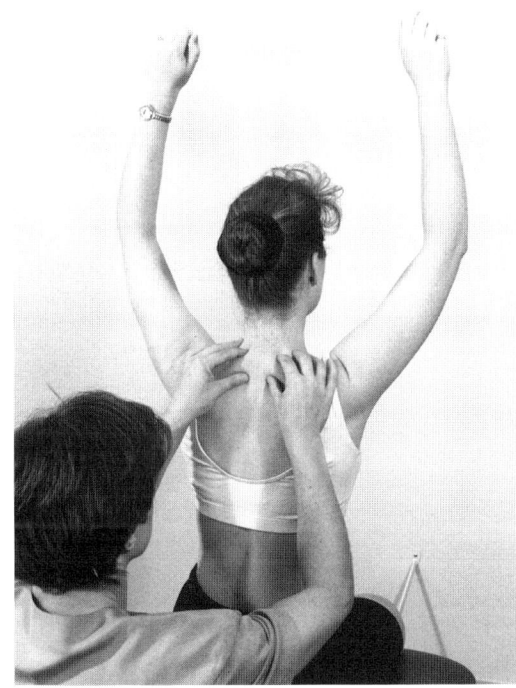

NOTES:

_____

_____

_____

_____

_____

ACTIVE MOBILITY TESTS OF OSTEOKINEMATIC FUNCTION — SPINAL

Lateral bending

Patient:	Sitting.
Therapist:	Standing behind the patient.
Palpate:	With the index finger and thumb of both hands, palpate the transverse processes of two adjacent vertebrae.
Test:	Instruct the patient to laterally bend the head and neck and note the quantity and direction of motion. When interpreting the mobility findings, the position of the joint at the beginning of the test should be correlated with the subsequent mobility noted, since alterations in joint mobility may merely be a reflection of an altered starting position.

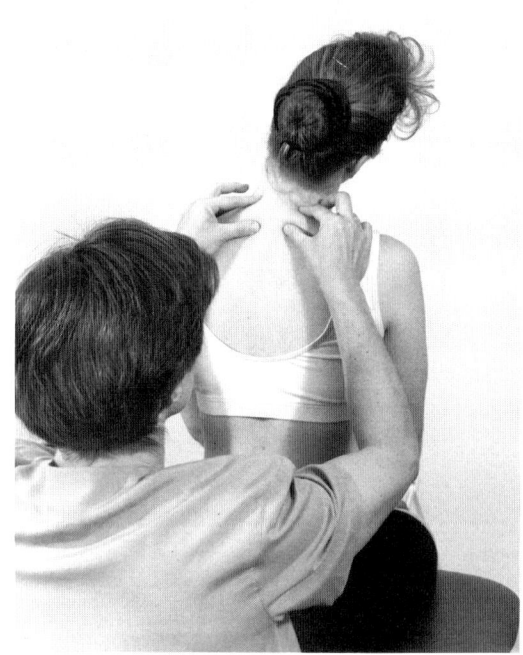

NOTES:

_____

_____

_____

_____

_____

_____

ACTIVE MOBILITY TESTS OF OSTEOKINEMATIC FUNCTION – SPINAL

Rotation

Patient: Sitting.
Therapist: Standing behind the patient.
Palpate: With the index finger and thumb of both hands, palpate the transverse processes of two adjacent vertebrae.
Test: Instruct the patient to rotate the head and neck and note the quantity and direction of motion. When interpreting the mobility findings, the position of the joint at the beginning of the test should be correlated with the subsequent mobility noted since alterations in joint mobility may merely be a reflection of an altered starting position.

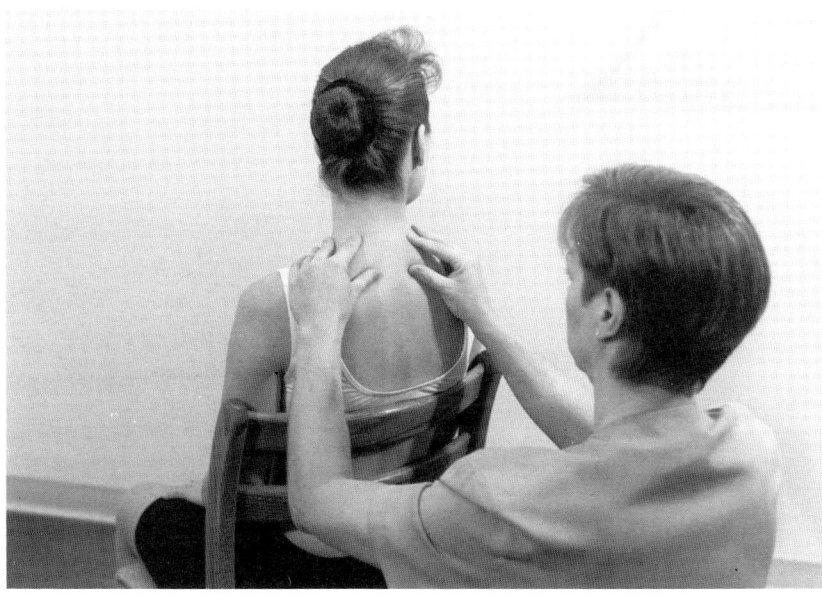

NOTES:

_____

_____

_____

_____

_____

_____

_____

_____

ACTIVE MOBILITY TESTS OF OSTEOKINEMATIC FUNCTION – COSTAL

Forward bending

Patient: Sitting.

Therapist: Standing behind the patient.

Palpate: With the thumb of one hand, palpate the rib just lateral to the tubercle and medial to the angle. The index finger of this hand rests along the shaft of the rib. With the thumb of the other hand, palpate the transverse process to which the rib attaches.

Test: Instruct the patient to forward bend the head and neck and note the quantity and direction of relative motion between the vertebra and the rib. When interpreting the mobility findings, the position of the joint at the beginning of the test should be correlated with the subsequent mobility noted since alterations in joint mobility may merely be a reflection of an altered starting position.

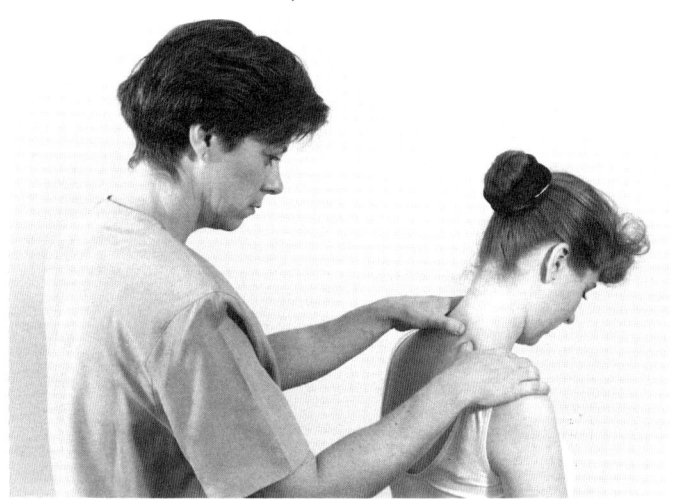
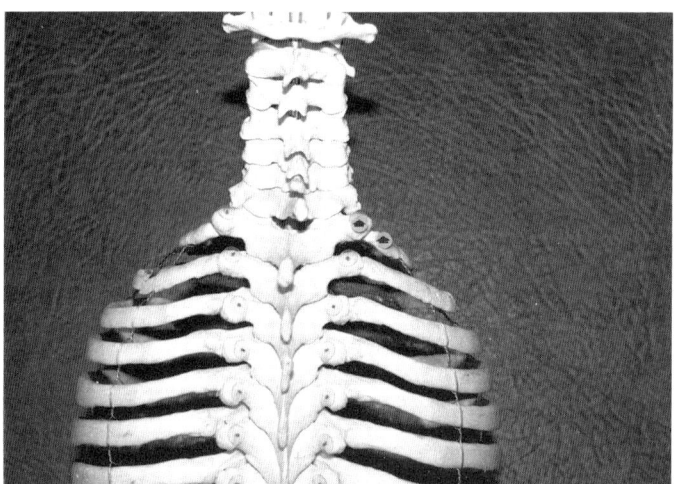

NOTES:

_____

_____

_____

_____

_____

_____

_____

ACTIVE MOBILITY TESTS OF OSTEOKINEMATIC FUNCTION — COSTAL

Backward bending

Patient:	Sitting.
Therapist:	Standing behind the patient.
Palpate:	With the thumb of one hand, palpate the rib just lateral to the tubercle and medial to the angle. The index finger of this hand rests along the shaft of the rib. With the thumb of the other hand, palpate the transverse process to which the rib attaches.
Test:	Instruct the patient to elevate both arms and note the quantity and direction of relative motion between the vertebra and the rib. Ensure that the shoulder girdles do not elevate and the head does not "poke forward"during this test. When interpreting the mobility findings, the position of the joint at the beginning of the test should be correlated with the subsequent mobility noted since alterations in joint mobility may merely be a reflection of an altered starting position.

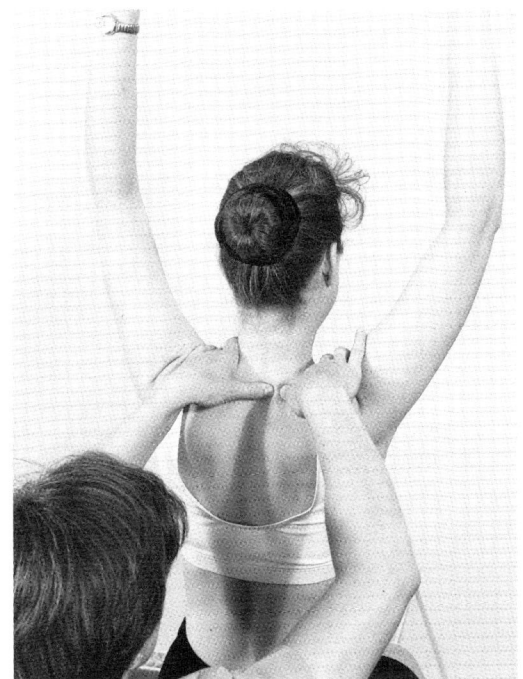

NOTES: _____

_____

_____

_____

ACTIVE MOBILITY TESTS OF OSTEOKINEMATIC FUNCTION — COSTAL

Lateral bending

Patient:	Sitting.
Therapist:	Standing behind the patient.
Palpate:	With the thumb of one hand, palpate the rib just lateral to the tubercle and medial to the angle. The index finger of this hand rests along the shaft of the rib. With the thumb of the other hand, palpate the transverse process to which the rib attaches.
Test:	Instruct the patient to laterally bend the head and neck and note the quantity and direction of relative motion between the vertebra and the rib. When interpreting the mobility findings, the position of the joint at the beginning of the test should be correlated with the subsequent mobility noted since alterations in joint mobility may merely be a reflection of an altered starting position.

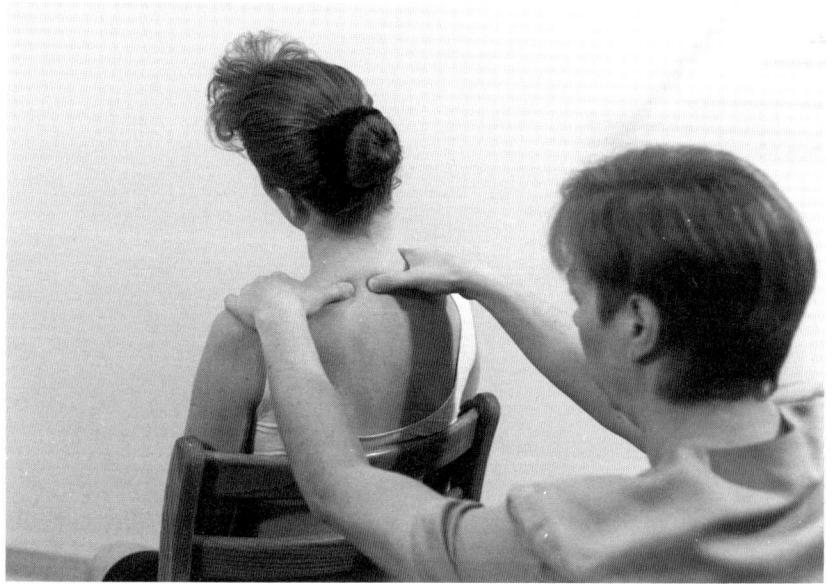

NOTES:

_____

_____

_____

_____

_____

_____

ACTIVE MOBILITY TESTS OF OSTEOKINEMATIC FUNCTION — COSTAL

Rotation

Patient:	Sitting.
Therapist:	Standing behind the patient.
Palpate:	With the thumb of one hand, palpate the rib just lateral to the tubercle and medial to the angle. The index finger of this hand rests along the shaft of the rib. With the thumb of the other hand, palpate the transverse process to which the rib attaches.
Test:	Instruct the patient to rotate the head and neck and note the quantity and direction of relative motion between the vertebra and the rib. When interpreting the mobility findings, the position of the joint at the beginning of the test should be correlated with the subsequent mobility noted since alterations in joint mobility may merely be a reflection of an altered starting position.

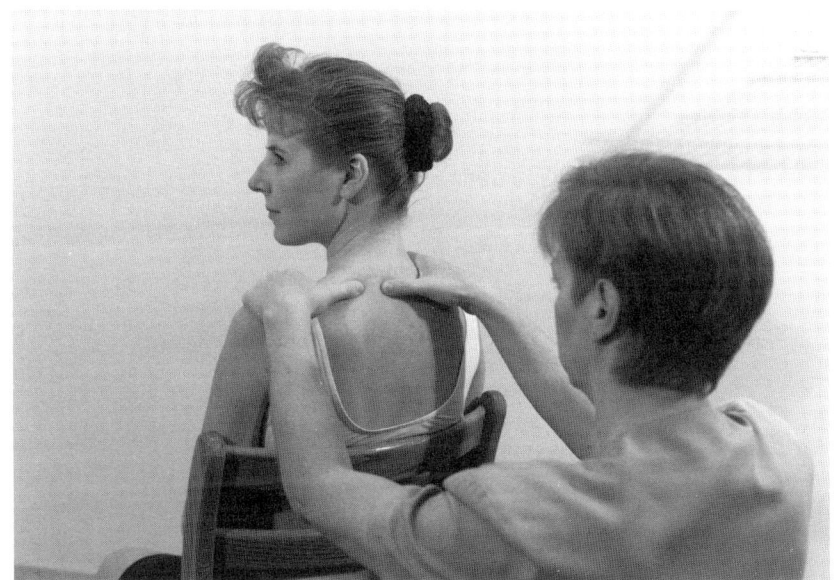

NOTES:

_____

_____

_____

_____

_____

_____

ACTIVE MOBILITY TESTS OF OSTEOKINEMATIC FUNCTION – COSTAL

Respiration

Patient: Sitting.

Dorsal Therapist: Standing behind the patient.

Palpate: With the thumb of one hand, palpate the rib just lateral to the tubercle and medial to the angle. The index finger of this hand rests along the shaft of the rib. With the thumb of the other hand, palpate the transverse process to which the rib attaches.

Test: Instruct the patient to take a deep breath in and note the quantity and direction of relative motion between the vertebra and the rib. Instruct the patient to breathe out and note the quantity and direction of relative motion between the vertebra and the rib. When interpreting the mobility findings, the position of the joint at the beginning of the test should be correlated with the subsequent mobility noted since alterations in joint mobility may merely be a reflection of an altered starting position.

NOTES:

_____

_____

_____

_____

ACTIVE MOBILITY TESTS OF OSTEOKINEMATIC FUNCTION — COSTAL

Respiration

Patient: Sitting.

Ventral Therapist: Standing in front of the patient.

Palpate: First rib - With the index fingers or thumbs, palpate the ventral aspect of the first ribs at the manubriocostal junction.

Second rib - With the index fingers or thumbs, palpate the superior aspect of the second ribs at the manubriocostal junction.

Test: Instruct the patient to take a deep breath in and note the quantity and symmetry of motion. Instruct the patient to breathe out and note the quantity and symmetry of motion. When interpreting the mobility findings, the position of the joint at the beginning of the test should be correlated with the subsequent mobility noted since alterations in joint mobility may merely be a reflection of an altered starting position.

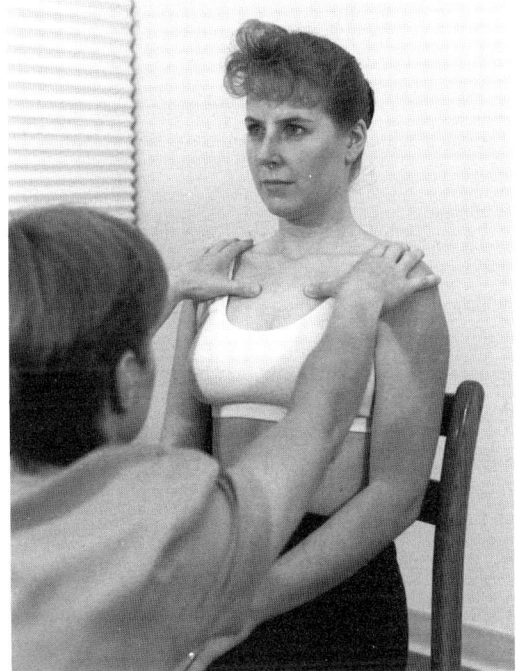

NOTES: _____

_____

_____

PASSIVE MOBILITY TESTS OF OSTEOKINEMATIC FUNCTION

Flexion/extension/lateral bending/rotation

Patient: Sitting.

Therapist: Standing at the patient's side.

Palpate: With the index finger of the dorsal hand, palpate the interspinous space of the segment being tested. The ulnar border of the fifth finger of the ventral hand palpates the lamina and inferior articular pillar of the cranial vertebra. The rest of this hand supports the cervical spine and the arm cradles the cranium.

Test: Passively flex, extend, laterally bend, rotate the segment and note the quantity, quality, direction of ease and the end feel of motion.

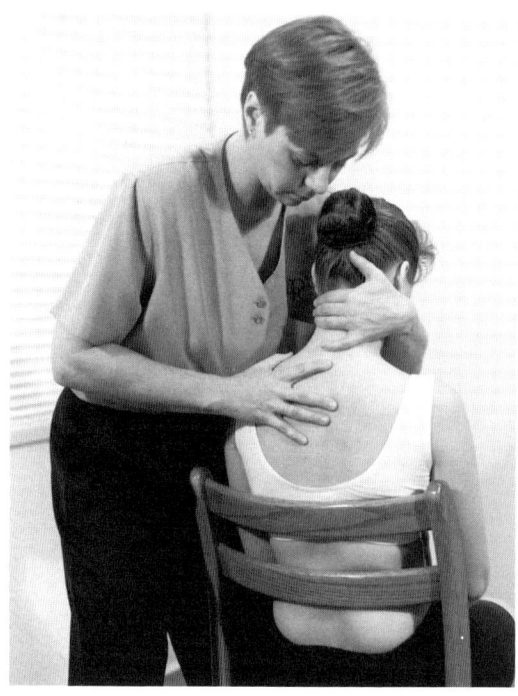

NOTES:

_____

_____

_____

_____

_____

_____

_____

PASSIVE MOBILITY TESTS OF ARTHROKINEMATIC FUNCTION – SPINAL

Superoanterior glide – right T1-2 zygapophysial joint

Patient:	Prone.
Therapist:	Standing at the patient's side.
Palpate:	With the left thumb, palpate the inferior aspect of the left transverse process of T2. With the right thumb, palpate the inferior aspect of the right transverse process of T1.
Test:	Fix T2 and apply a force, varying the mediolateral inclination, to produce a superoanterior glide (arrow) of the right zygapophysial joint at T1-2 with the right thumb. Note the quantity, direction of ease and the end feel of motion.

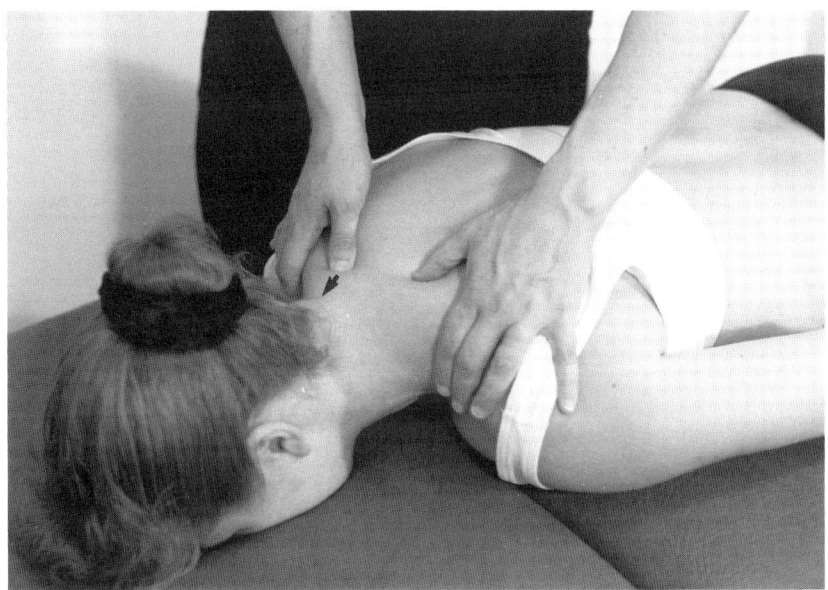

NOTES:

_____

_____

_____

_____

_____

_____

_____

_____

PASSIVE MOBILITY TESTS OF ARTHROKINEMATIC FUNCTION – SPINAL

Inferoposterior glide – right T1-2 zygapophysial joint

Patient:	Prone.
Therapist:	Standing at the patient's side.
Palpate:	With the left thumb, palpate the inferior aspect of the right transverse process of T2. With the right thumb, palpate the superior aspect of the right transverse process of T1.
Test:	Fix T2 with an anterosuperior pressure and apply a force, varying the mediolateral inclination, to produce an inferoposterior glide (arrow) of the zygapophysial joint at T1-2 with the right thumb. Note the quantity, direction of ease and the end feel of motion.

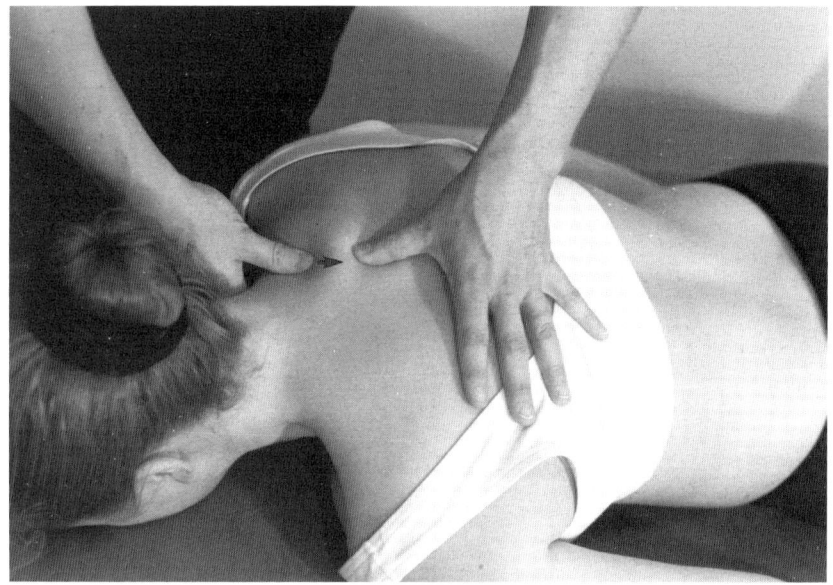

NOTES:

_____

_____

_____

_____

_____

_____

_____

_____

PASSIVE MOBILITY TESTS OF ARTHROKINEMATIC FUNCTION – COSTAL

Superior glide/anterior roll – right first costotransverse joint

Patient:	Supine.
Therapist:	Standing at the patient's head facing the shoulders.
Palpate:	With the right thumb, palpate the superior aspect of the right transverse process of T1. With the index and long finger, palpate the inferior aspect of the right first rib.
Test:	Fix the right first rib with the right index and long finger and apply a force to the transverse process of T1 with the thumb to produce a posteroinferor glide (black arrow) of the right first costotransverse joint. This motion produces a relative superior glide/anterior roll of the first rib at the costotranverse joint. Note the quantity, direction of ease and the end feel of motion.

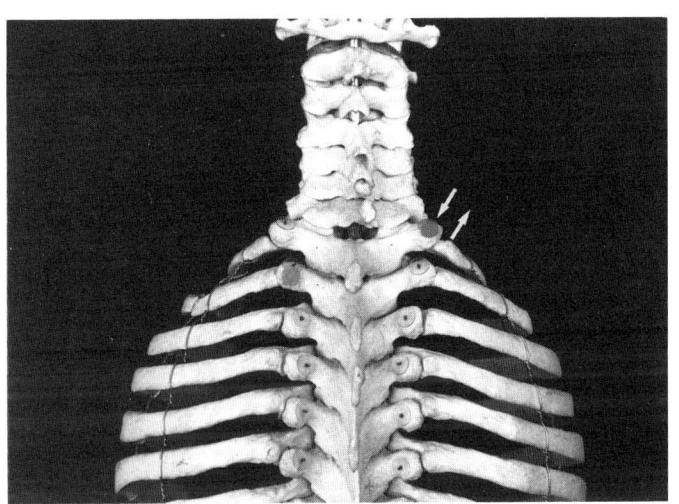
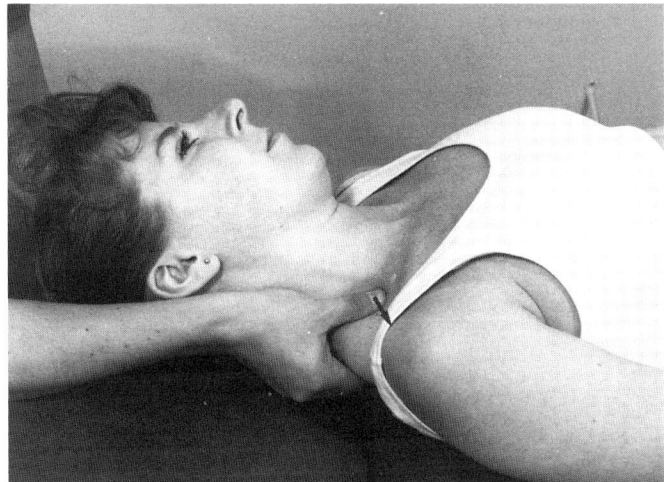

NOTES:

_____

_____

_____

_____

_____

_____

_____

_____

_____

PASSIVE MOBILITY TESTS OF ARTHROKINEMATIC FUNCTION – COSTAL

Inferior glide/posterior roll – right first costotransverse joint

Patient: Supine.
Therapist: Standing at the patient's head facing the shoulders.
Palpate: With the radial aspect of the MCP joint of the index finger of the left hand, palpate and fix the superior aspect of the left transverse process of T1. With the radial aspect of the MCP joint of the index finger of the right hand, palpate the superior aspect of the right first rib just lateral to the costotransverse joint.
Test: Fix T1 and apply a force to produce an inferoanterior glide (arrow) of the right first costotransverse joint. Allow the conjunct posterior roll to occur. Note the quantity, direction of ease and the end feel of motion.

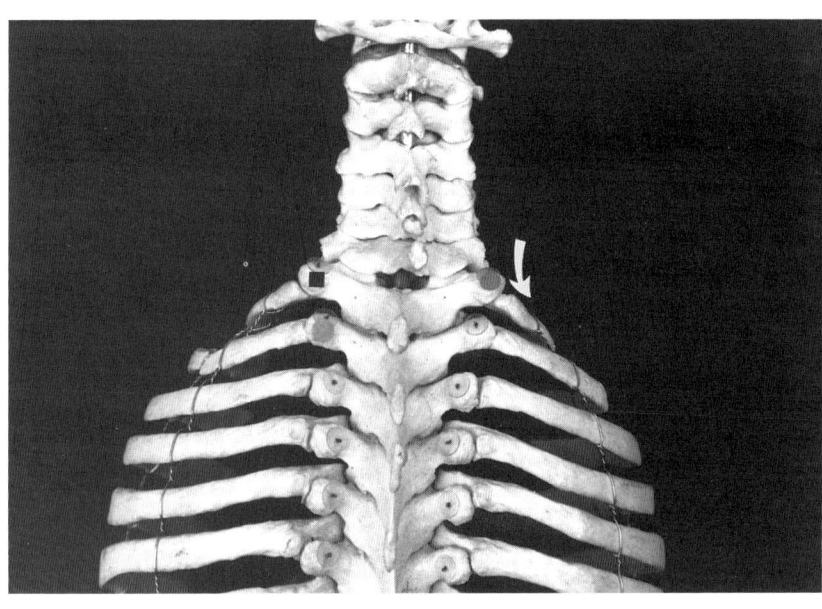
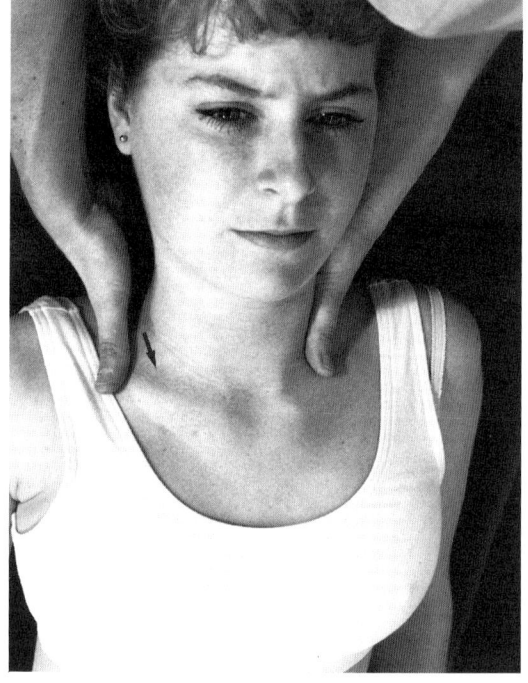

NOTES:

_____

_____

_____

_____

_____

_____

PASSIVE STABILITY TESTS OF ARTHROKINETIC FUNCTION – SPINAL

Vertical (traction)

Patient: Sitting.
Therapist: Standing behind the patient.
Palpate: With both thumbs, palpate the posteroinferior aspect of the occiput. The rest of the hand is applied to the lateral aspect of the cranium.
Test: Apply a vertical traction force (arrow) to the cervicothoracic junction through the head and neck. The region may be localized by varying the degree of flexion of the head and neck. The force is sustained for 20 seconds. Note the reproduction of any symptoms.

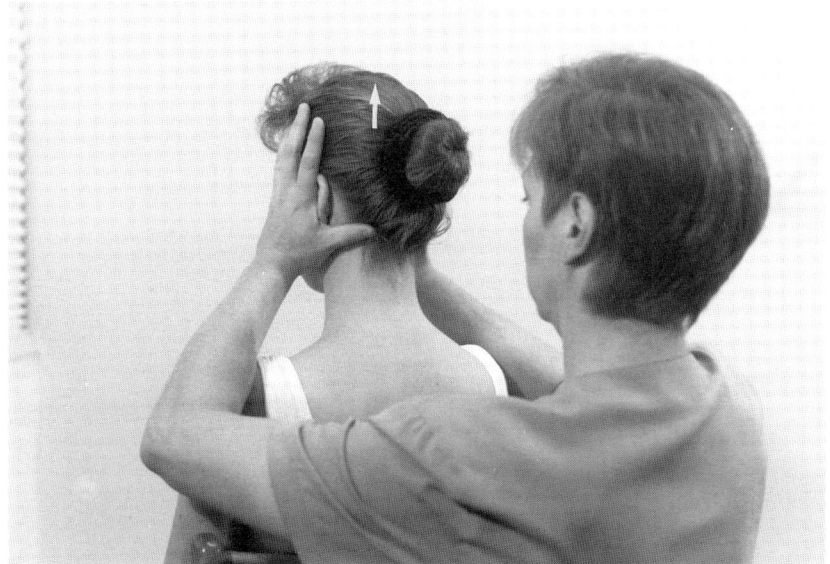

NOTES:

_____

_____

_____

_____

_____

_____

_____

_____

_____

_____

PASSIVE STABILITY TESTS OF ARTHROKINETIC FUNCTION – SPINAL

Vertical (Compression)

Patient: Sitting.
Therapist: Standing behind the patient.
Palpate: With both hands, palpate the top of the head.
Test: Apply a vertical compression force (arrow) to the cervicothoracic junction through the head and neck. The force is sustained for 20 seconds. Note the reproduction of any symptoms.

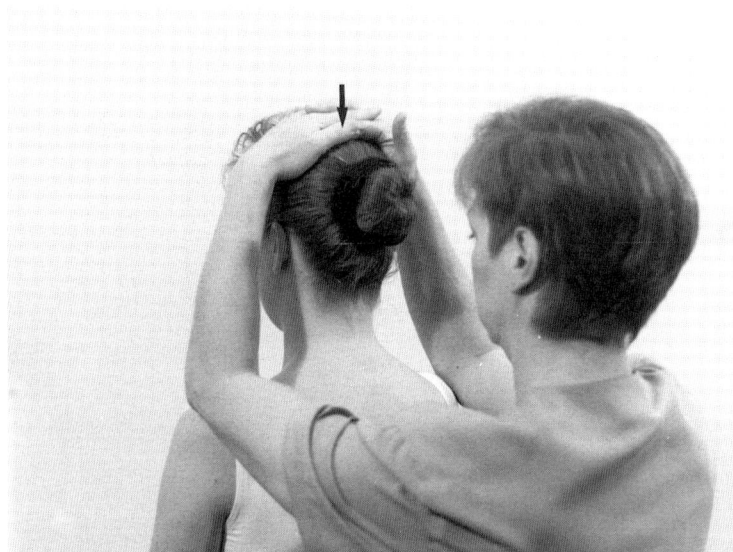

NOTES:

_____

_____

_____

_____

_____

_____

_____

_____

_____

_____

PASSIVE STABILITY TESTS OF ARTHROKINETIC FUNCTION – SPINAL

Anterior translation

Patient: Prone.
Therapist: Standing at the patient's side.
Palpate: With one hand, palpate the transverse processes of the cranial vertebra. With the other hand, palpate the transverse processes of the caudal vertebra.
Test: Apply an anterior translation force (arrow) through the cranial vertebra while fixing the caudal vertebra. Sustain the force until the end feel is perceived. Note the quantity of motion, the reproduction of any symptoms and the end feel of motion.

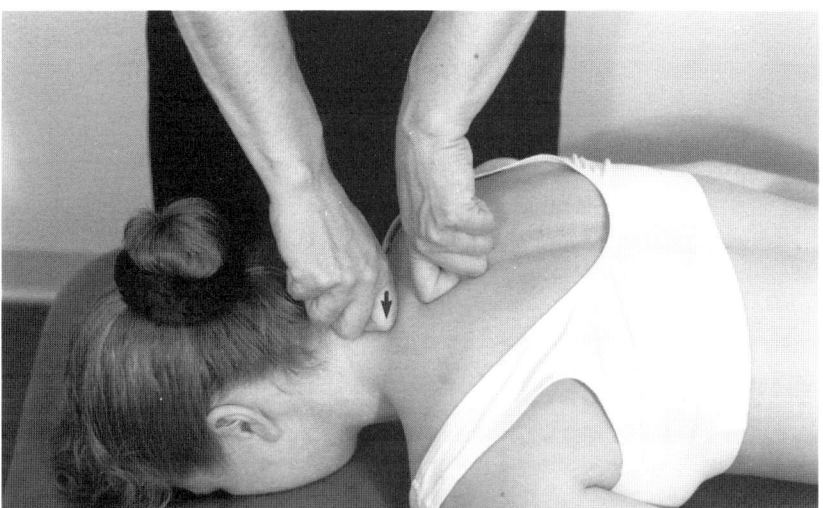

NOTES:

_____

_____

_____

_____

_____

_____

_____

_____

PASSIVE STABILITY TESTS OF ARTHROKINETIC FUNCTION – SPINAL

Posterior translation

Patient: Supine, shoulders supported on the table, head and neck supported by the therapist.

Therapist: Standing at the patient's head facing the shoulders.

Palpate: With the radial aspect of the index finger of one hand, palpate transversely the caudal vertebra of the segment being tested. With the other hand, support the head and neck such that the index finger supports the cranial vertebra of the segment being tested.

Test: Apply a posterior translation force (arrow) through the cranial vertebra while fixing the caudal vertebra. Sustain the force until the end feel is perceived. Note the quantity of motion, the reproduction of any symptoms and the end feel of motion.

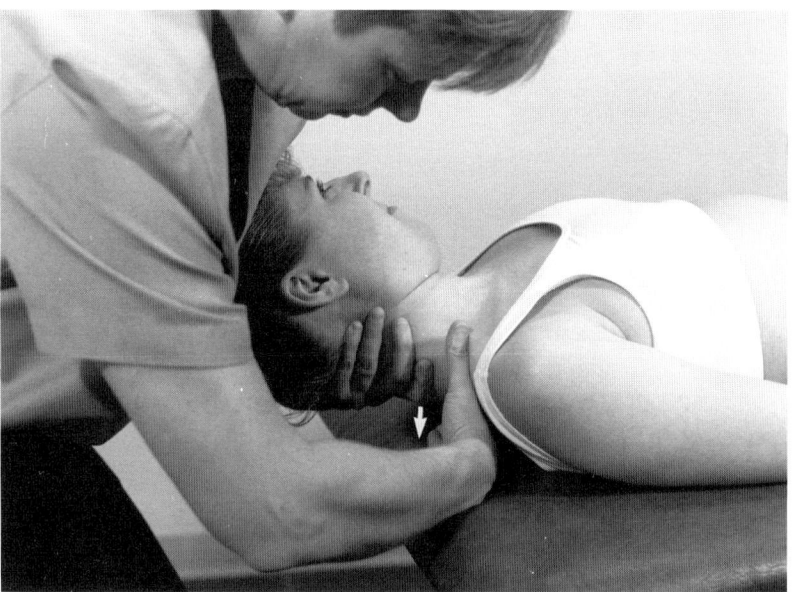

NOTES:

_____

_____

_____

_____

_____

_____

_____

PASSIVE STABILITY TESTS OF ARTHROKINETIC FUNCTION — SPINAL

Rotation

Patient:	Prone.
Therapist:	Standing at the patient's side.
Palpate:	With one hand, palpate the transverse process of the cranial vertebra. With the other hand, palpate the transverse process of the caudal vertebra on the contralateral side.
Test:	Fix the caudal vertebra and apply a posteroanterior force (arrow) through the cranial vertebra. Sustain the force until the end feel is perceived. Note the quantity of motion, the reproduction of any symptoms and the end feel of motion.

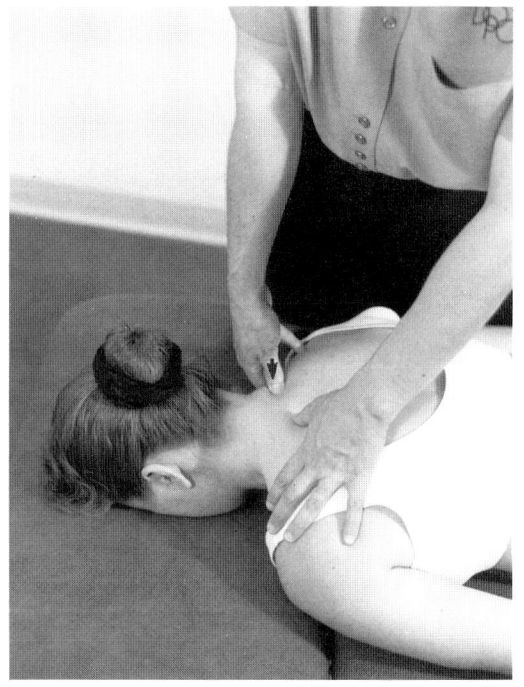

NOTES:

_____

_____

_____

_____

_____

_____

_____

PASSIVE STABILITY TESTS OF ARTHROKINETIC FUNCTION – COSTAL

Anterior translation – posterior aspect

Patient:	Prone.
Therapist:	Standing at the patient's side.
Palpate:	With one hand, fix the contralateral transverse processes of the vertebrae to which the rib attaches. For example, when testing the right second rib, the left transverse processes of T1 and T2 are fixed. With the other hand, palpate the rib just lateral to the tubercle.
Test:	Apply a posteroanterior force (arrow) to the rib while fixing the thoracic vertebrae. Sustain the force until the end feel is perceived. Note the quantity of motion, the reproduction of any symptoms and the end feel of motion.

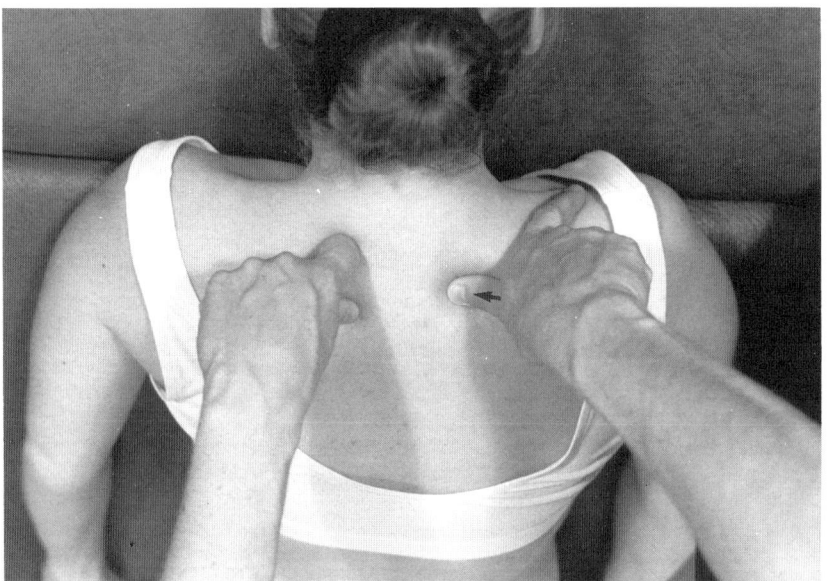

NOTES:

_____

_____

_____

_____

_____

_____

_____

_____

PASSIVE STABILITY TESTS OF ARTHROKINETIC FUNCTION – COSTAL

Anteroposterior translation – sternochondral/costochondral

Patient: Supine, head supported on a pillow.

Therapist: Standing at the patient's side.

Palpate: With one thumb, palpate the anterior aspect of the manubrium/costal cartilage. With the other thumb, palpate the anterior aspect of the costal cartilage/rib.

Test: Apply an anteroposterior force to the:
a) manubrium (manubriocostal junction)
b) sternal end of the costal cartilage (manubriocostal junction)
c) costal end of the costal cartilage (costochondral junction)
d) cartilagenous end of the rib (costochondral junction).

Sustain the force until the end feel is perceived. Note the quantity of motion, the reproduction of any symptoms and the end feel of motion.

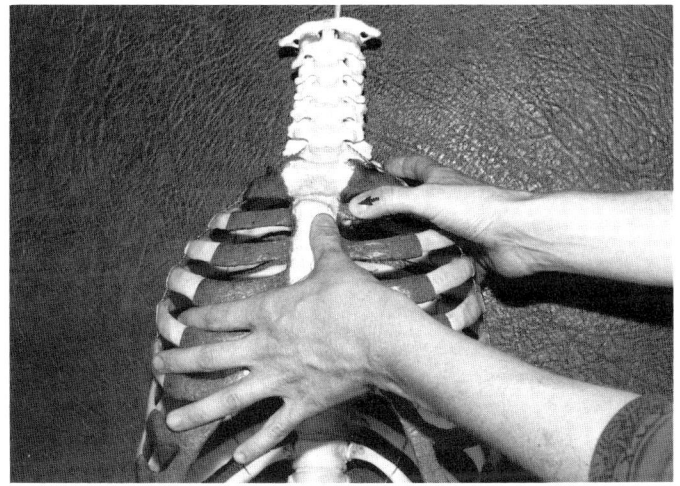 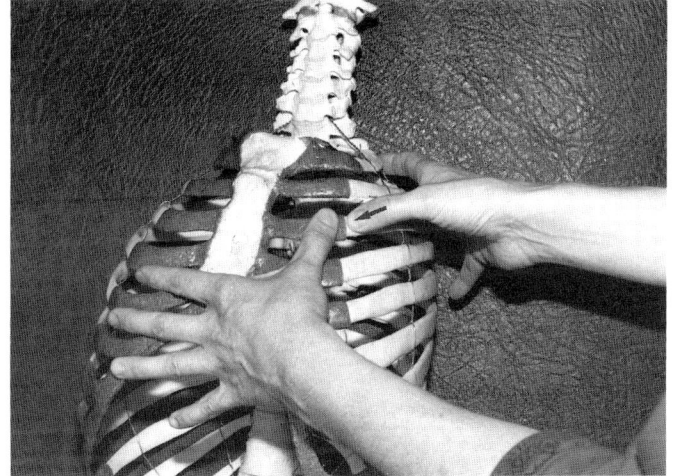

NOTES:

_____

_____

_____

_____

_____

_____

_____

PASSIVE STABILITY TESTS OF ARTHROKINETIC FUNCTION — COSTAL

Superoinferior translation – sternochondral/costochondral

Patient:	Supine, head supported on a pillow.
Therapist:	Standing at the patient's side.
Palpate:	With one thumb, palpate the superior aspect of the manubrium/costal cartilage. With the other thumb, palpate the inferior aspect of the costal cartilage/rib.
Test:	Apply a superoinferior force to the:

a) manubrium (manubriocostal junction)

b) sternal end of the costal cartilage (manubriocostal junction)

c) costal end of the costal cartilage (costochondral junction)

d) cartilagenous end of the rib (costochondral junction).

Sustain the force until the end feel is perceived. Note the quantity of motion, the reproduction of any symptoms and the end feel of motion.

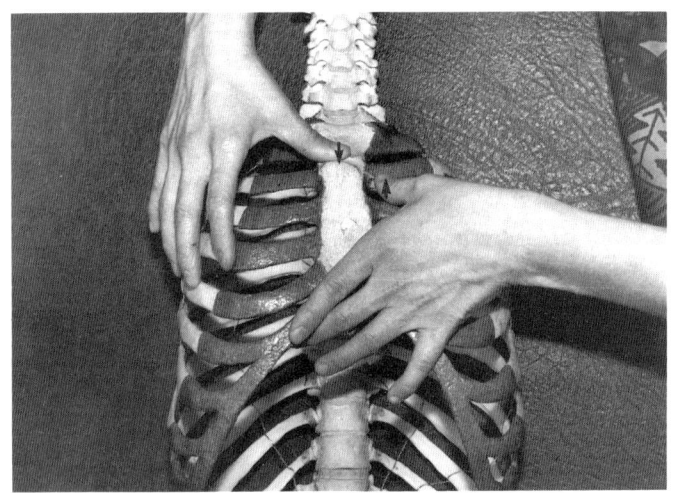 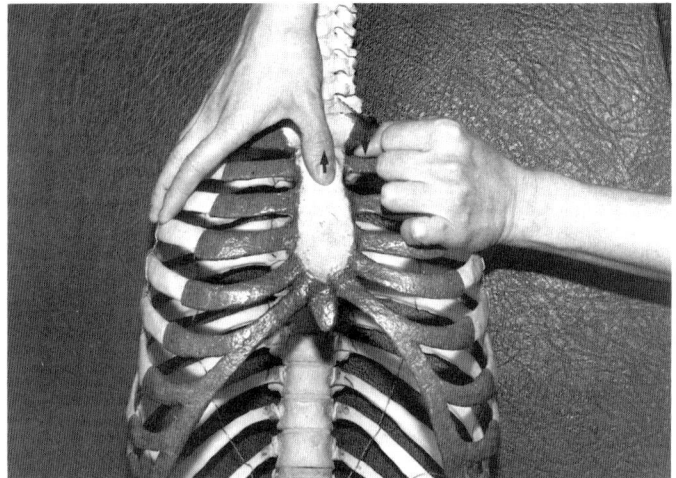

NOTES:

_____

_____

_____

_____

_____

_____

_____

MOBILIZATION TECHNIQUES — SPINAL

Traction

Supine
Patient:	Supine.
Therapist:	Standing at the patient's head facing the shoulders.
Palpate:	With the radial aspect of the index finger, palpate the interspinous space at the level being treated. With an open pinch grip of the other hand, palpate the cranial vertebra of the segment being treated. The rest of this hand supports the head and neck.
Localization:	Flex or extend the segment until the neutral position is achieved.
Mobilization:	Grade 1 to 4 traction is applied by fixing the caudal vertebra and pulling the cranial vertebra superiorly.

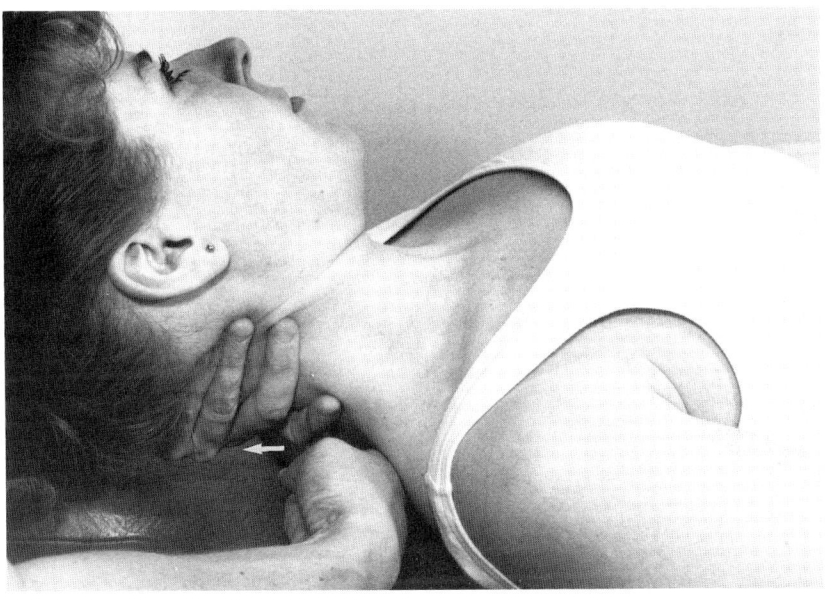

NOTES:

_____

_____

_____

_____

_____

_____

_____

MOBILIZATION TECHNIQUES — SPINAL

Traction

Sitting

Patient: Sitting, hands placed behind the neck with the fingers interlaced.

Therapist: Standing behind the patient.

Palpate: Wind both arms under the patient's axillae and place the hands over the patient's interlaced fingers on the back of the neck. Gently grip the thorax under the axillae with the inner arms.

Mobilization: Instruct the patient to look forward in order to relax the ligamentum nuche. Grade 1 to 5 traction is applied by rocking the patient back and up, allowing gravity to traction the joint.

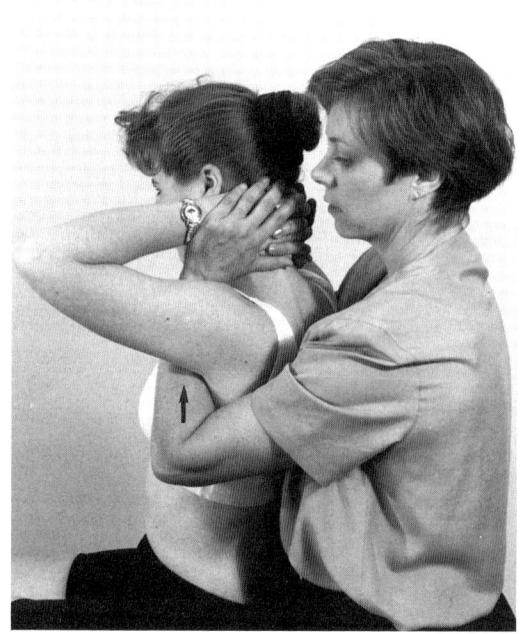

NOTES:

_____

_____

_____

_____

_____

_____

MOBILIZATION TECHNIQUES — SPINAL

Restriction of flexion/left lateral bending/rotation (superoanterior glide) – right T1-2 zygapophysial joint

Supine

Patient:	Supine.
Therapist:	Standing at the patient's head facing the shoulders.
Palpate:	With the radial aspect of the left index finger, palpate the left transverse process of T1. With the other hand, support the midcervical spine down to C7.
Localization:	Stabilise C7-T1 by laterally bending C7-T1 to the left and rotating it to the right. Localize T1-2 by flexing T1-2 and then gliding the left transverse process of T1 inferomedially on T2.
Mobilization:	**Passive** – With the left hand, apply a grade 1 to 5 force to produce an inferomedial and slightly posterior glide of the left zygapophysial joint at T1-2 (arrow). This will mobilize the right zygapophysial joint of T1-2 into flexion by producing a superior and slightly anterior glide of the right zygapophysial joint at T1-2.
	Active – From the motion barrier, instruct the patient to resist further motion and apply a gentle force to the head/neck. The direction of this force is that which facilitates flexion/left lateral bending/rotation. The isometric contraction is held for up to 5 seconds and followed by a period of complete relaxation. The joint is then passively taken to the new motion barrier. This technique is repeated 3 times and followed by a re-evaluation of osteokinematic, arthrokinematic and arthrokinetic function.

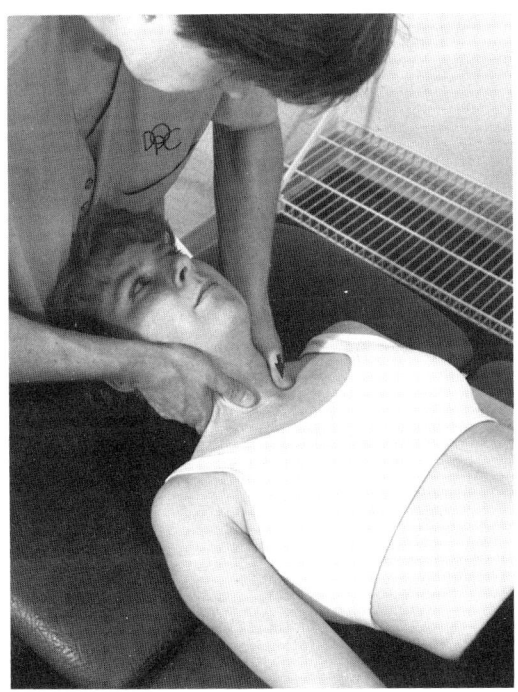

MOBILIZATION TECHNIQUES — SPINAL

Restriction of flexion/left lateral bending/rotation – T1-2

Sitting

Patient: Sitting, spine supported against the chair.

Therapist: Standing at the patient's side.

Palpate: With the dorsal hand, fix the caudal vertebra by applying pressure to the spinous process with the thumb. The ulnar border of the ring or fifth finger of the ventral hand is applied to the lamina and inferior articular process, or hooked around the spinous process, of the cranial vertebra.

Mobilization: **Passive** – Apply a grade 1 to 4 force to produce a superoanterior glide (arrow) of the right zygapophysial joint at T1-2.

Active – From the motion barrier, instruct the patient to resist further motion and apply a gentle force to the head/neck. The direction of this force is that which facilitates flexion/left lateral bending/rotation at T1-2. The isometric contraction is held for up to 5 seconds and followed by a period of complete relaxation. The joint is then passively taken to the new motion barrier. This technique is repeated 3 times and followed by a re-evaluation of osteokinematic, arthrokinematic and arthrokinetic function.

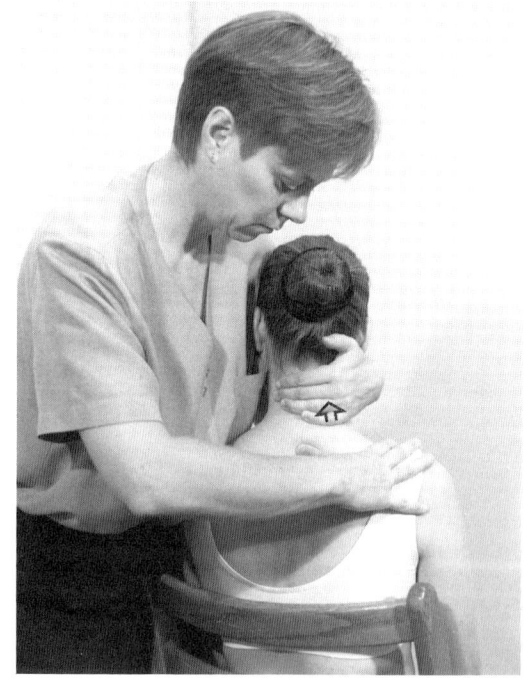

MOBILIZATION TECHNIQUES – SPINAL

Restriction of extension (inferoposterior glide) – zygapophyseal joints

Patient:	Supine, shoulders supported on the table, head and neck supported by the therapist.
Therapist:	Standing at the patient's head facing the shoulders.
Palpate:	With the radial aspect of the index finger, palpate transversely the interspinous space of the segment. Support the lower cervical spine and head with the other hand.
Mobilization:	**Passive** – Apply a grade 1 to 4 force to produce a posteroinferior glide of the zygapophyseal joints of the segment (arrow).
	Active – From the motion barrier, instruct the patient to hold the head still while support is minimally released. The isometric contraction is held for up to 5 seconds and followed by a period of complete relaxation. The joint is then passively taken to the new motion barrier. This technique is repeated 3 times and followed by a re-evaluation of osteokinematic, arthrokinematic and arthrokinetic function.

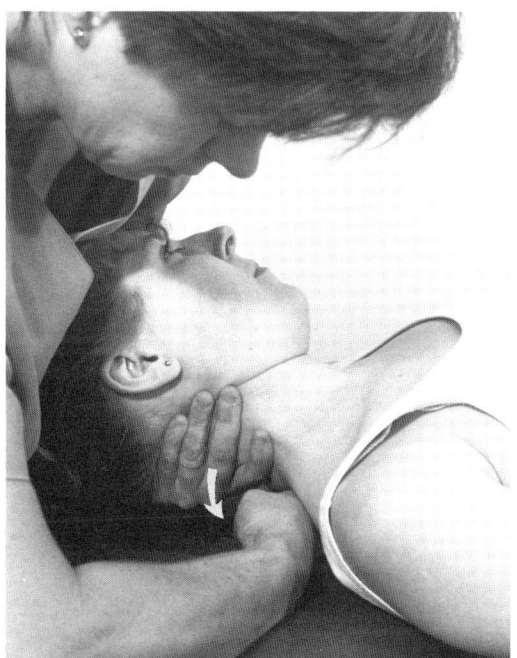

NOTES:

_____

_____

_____

MOBILIZATION TECHNIQUES – SPINAL

Restriction of extension/right lateral bending/rotation (inferoposteromedial glide) – right T1-2 zygapophysial joint

Patient:	Supine.
Therapist:	Standing at the patient's head facing the shoulders.
Palpate:	With the radial aspect of the right index finger, palpate the right transverse process of T1. With the other hand, support the head and neck.
Localization:	Stabilise C7-T1 by laterally bending C7-T1 to the right and rotating it to the left. Localize T1-2 by extending T1-2 and then gliding the right transverse process of T1 inferoposteromedially on T2.
Mobilization:	**Passive** – With the right hand, apply a grade 1 to 5 force to produce an inferoposteromedial glide (arrow) of the right zygapophysial joint at T1-2.
	Active – From the motion barrier, instruct the patient to resist further motion and apply a gentle force to the head/neck. The direction of this force is that which facilitates extension/right lateral bending/rotation. The isometric contraction is held for up to 5 seconds and followed by a period of complete relaxation. The joint is then passively taken to the new motion barrier. This technique is repeated 3 times and followed by a re-evaluation of osteokinematic, arthrokinematic and arthrokinetic function.

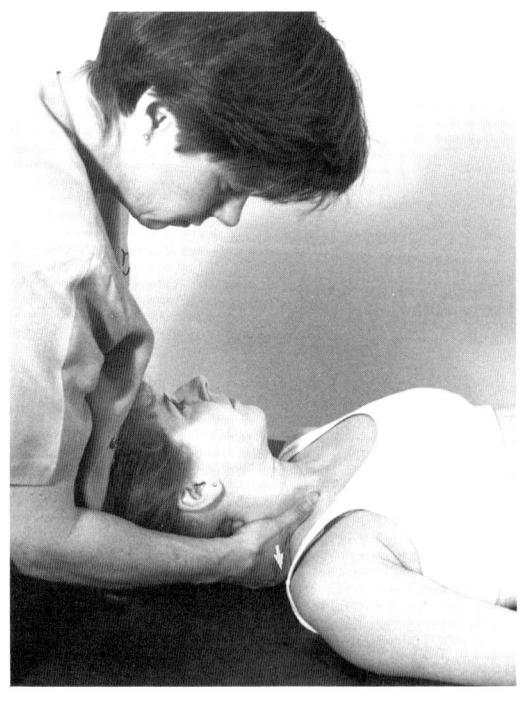

MOBILIZATION TECHNIQUES — COSTAL

Restriction of anterior rotation (superior glide/anterior roll) – right first costotransverse joint

Patient:	Supine.
Therapist:	Standing at the patient's head facing the shoulders.
Palpate:	With the right thumb, palpate the superior aspect of the right transverse process of T1. With the index and long finger of the right hand, palpate the inferior aspect of the right first rib. The other hand supports the midcervical spine.
Mobilization:	**Passive** – With the right thumb, apply a grade 1 to 4 force to the transverse process of T1 to produce a posteroinferior glide of the right transverse process. This will produce a relative superior glide/anterior roll of the first rib at the costotransverse joint.
	Active – From the motion barrier, instruct the patient to slowly breathe out. The joint is then passively taken to the new motion barrier. This technique is repeated 3 times and followed by a re-evaluation of osteokinematic, arthrokinematic and arthrokinetic function.

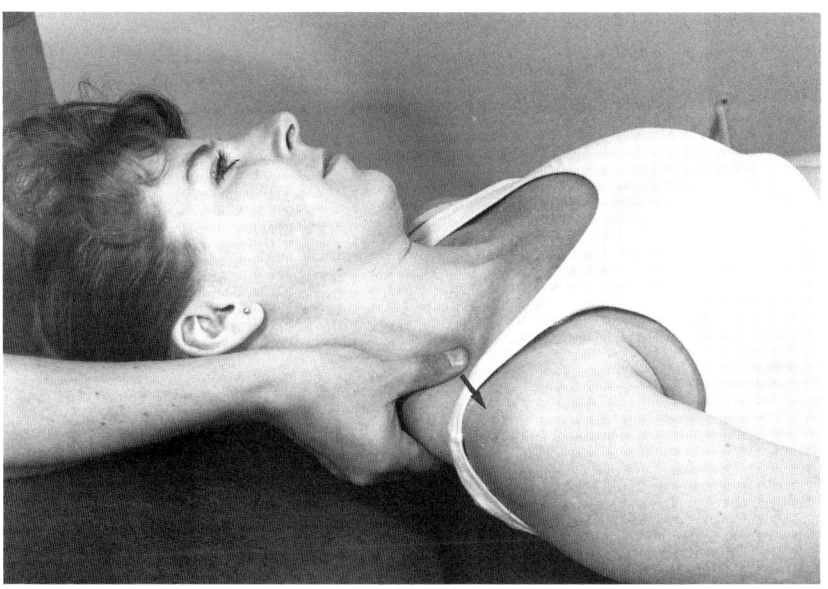

NOTES:

_____

_____

_____

_____

MOBILIZATION TECHNIQUES – COSTAL

Restriction of posterior rotation (inferior glide/posterior roll) – right first costotransverse joint

Patient: Supine.

Therapist: Standing at the patient's head facing the shoulders.

Palpate: With the radial aspect of the index finger of the right hand, palpate the superior aspect of the right first rib. The other hand supports the head and neck.

Localization: Stabilise C7-T1 and T1-2 by lateral bending to the right and rotation to the left. This is achieved with the left hand.

Mobilization: **Passive** – With the right hand, apply a grade 1 to 5 force to produce an anteroinferior glide (arrow) of the right first costotransverse joint. Allow the conjunct posterior roll to occur.

Active – From the motion barrier, instruct the patient to take a deep breath in. Following a period of complete relaxation, the joint is passively taken to the new motion barrier. This technique is repeated 3 times and followed by a re-evaluation of osteokinematic, arthrokinematic and arthrokinetic function.

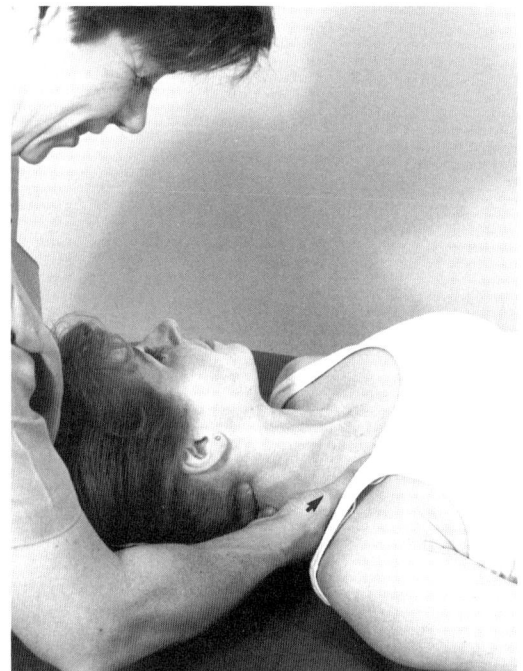

NOTES:

_____

_____

_____

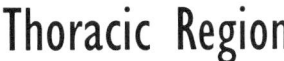

Thoracic Region

THORACIC REGION

ASSESSMENT

TREATMENT

POSITIONAL TESTS — SPINAL

Patient: Sitting.

Therapist: Standing behind the patient.

Palpate: With the thumbs, palpate the transverse processes of the T5 vertebra.

Test: **a)** Flex the joint complex and assess the position of T5 relative to T6 by noting which transverse process is the most dorsal. A dorsal left transverse process of T5 relative to T6 is indicative of a left rotated position of the T5-6 joint complex in flexion.

b) Extend the joint complex and assess the position of the T5 vertebra relative to T6 by noting which transverse process is the most dorsal. A dorsal left transverse process of T5 relative to T6 is indicative of a left rotated position of the T5-6 joint complex in extension.

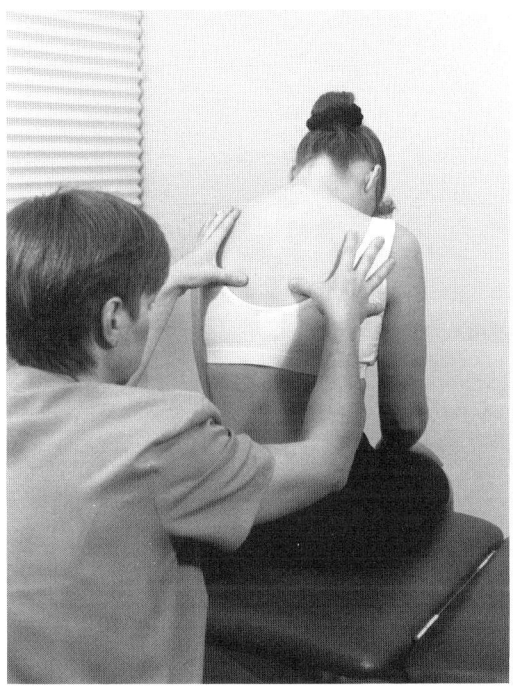

NOTES:

_____

_____

_____

_____

_____

_____

POSITIONAL TESTS — COSTAL

Dorsal

Patient:	Prone.
Therapist:	Standing at the patient's side.
Palpate:	With the thumbs, palpate the ribs just lateral to the tubercle and medial to the angle.
Test:	Note the craniocaudal, ventrodorsal relationship of the two ribs, left and right.

Ventral

Patient:	Supine.
Therapist:	Standing at the patient's side.
Palpate:	With the index fingers, palpate the ribs at the sternochondral junction.
Test:	Note the craniocaudal, ventrodorsal relationship of the two ribs, left and right.

Lateral

Patient:	Supine.
Therapist:	Standing at the patient's side.
Palpate:	With the index fingers, palpate the intercostal space and the lateral aspect of the ribs in the midaxillary line.
Test:	Note the distance between the two ribs and the prominence of the superior or inferior borders.

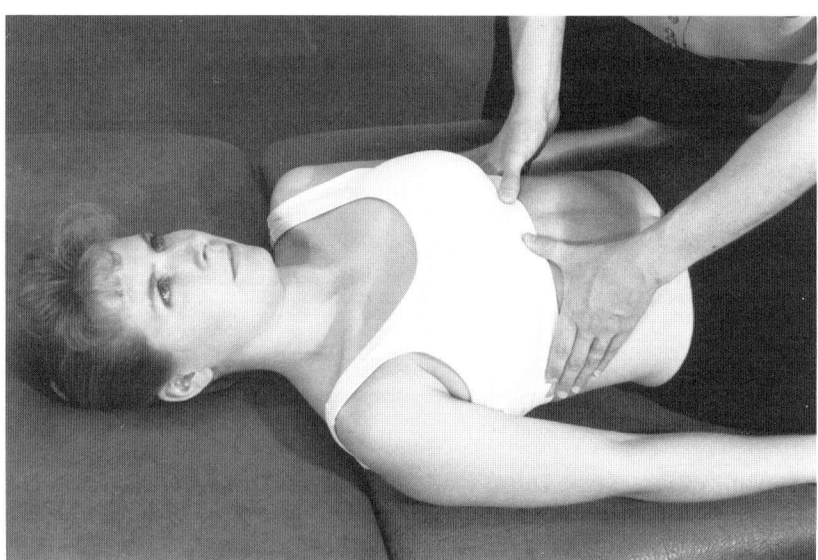

NOTES:

_____

_____

_____

_____

ACTIVE MOBILITY TESTS OF OSTEOKINEMATIC FUNCTION — SPINAL

Forward bending

Patient:	Sitting.
Therapist:	Standing behind the patient.
Palpate:	With the index finger and thumb of both hands, palpate the transverse processes of two adjacent vertebrae.
Test:	Instruct the patient to forward bend the thorax and note the quantity of motion as well as the symmetry of motion during flexion. Both index fingers should travel superiorly an equal distance. When interpreting the mobility findings, the position of the joint at the beginning of the test should be correlated with the subsequent mobility noted since alterations in joint mobility may merely be a reflection of an altered starting position.

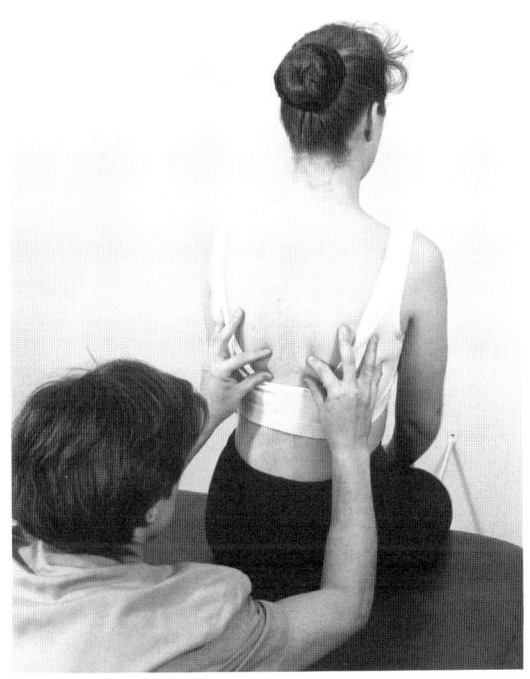
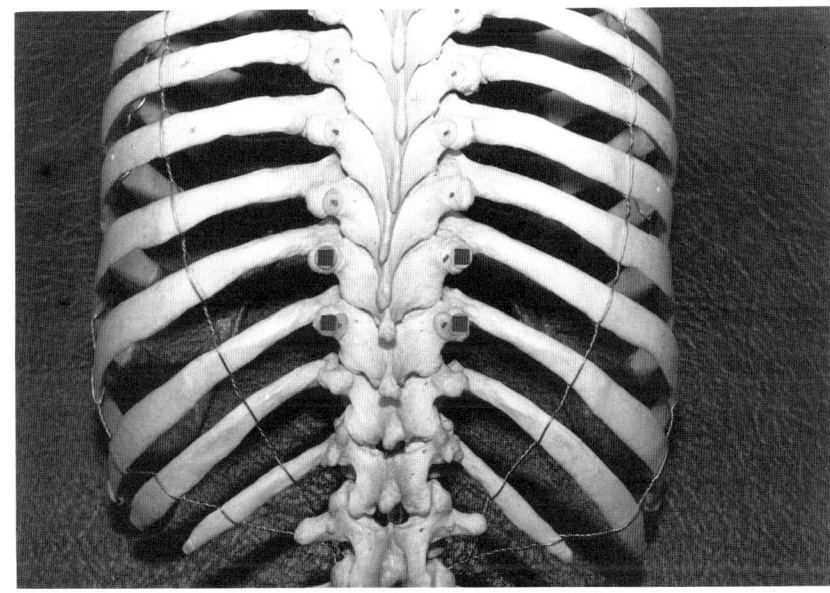

NOTES:

_____

_____

_____

_____

_____

ACTIVE MOBILITY TESTS OF OSTEOKINEMATIC FUNCTION – SPINAL

Backward bending

Patient: Sitting.
Therapist: Standing behind the patient.
Palpate: With the index finger and thumb of both hands, palpate the transverse processes of two adjacent vertebrae.
Test: Instruct the patient to backward bend the trunk and note the quantity of motion as well as the symmetry of motion during extension. Both index fingers should travel inferiorly an equal distance. When interpreting the mobility findings, the position of the joint at the beginning of the test should be correlated with the subsequent mobility noted since alterations in joint mobility may merely be a reflection of an altered starting position.

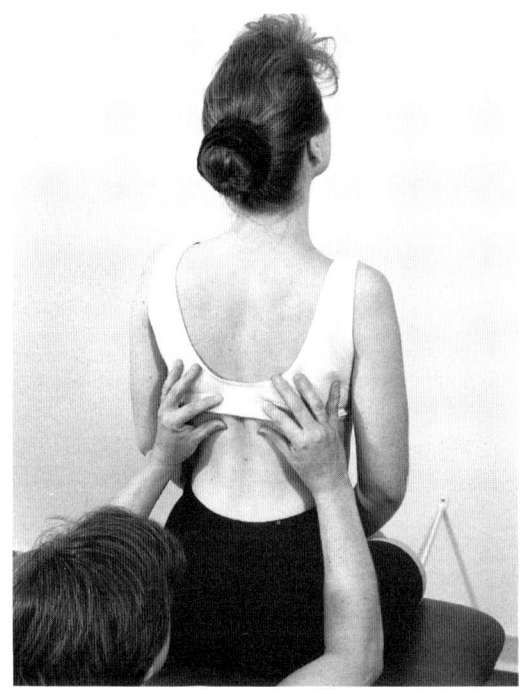

NOTES:

_____

_____

_____

_____

_____

ACTIVE MOBILITY TESTS OF OSTEOKINEMATIC FUNCTION — SPINAL

Lateral bending

Patient: Sitting.
Therapist: Standing behind the patient.
Palpate: With the index finger and thumb of both hands, palpate the transverse processes of two adjacent vertebrae.
Test: Instruct the patient to laterally bend the trunk and note the quantity and direction of motion. When interpreting the mobility findings, the position of the joint at the beginning of the test should be correlated with the subsequent mobility noted, since alterations in joint mobility may merely be a reflection of an altered starting position.

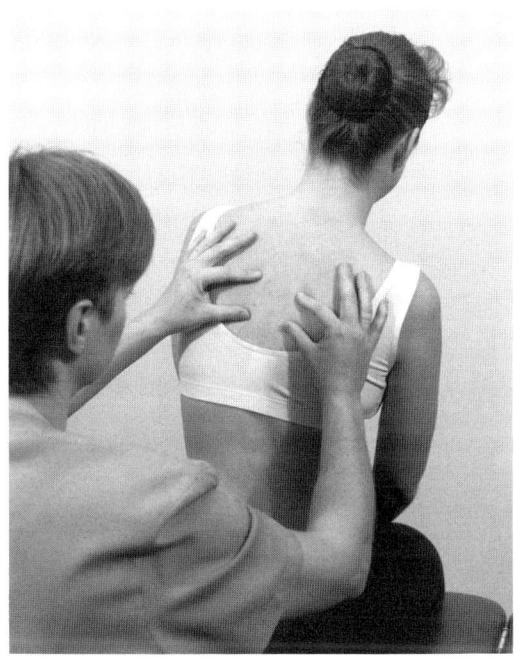

NOTES:

_____

_____

_____

_____

_____

_____

_____

ACTIVE MOBILITY TESTS OF OSTEOKINEMATIC FUNCTION – SPINAL

Rotation

Patient: Sitting.
Therapist: Standing behind the patient.
Palpate: With the index finger and thumb of both hands, palpate the transverse processes of two adjacent vertebrae.
Test: Instruct the patient to rotate the trunk and note the quantity and direction of motion. When interpreting the mobility findings, the position of the joint at the beginning of the test should be correlated with the subsequent mobility noted, since alterations in joint mobility may merely be a reflection of an altered starting position.

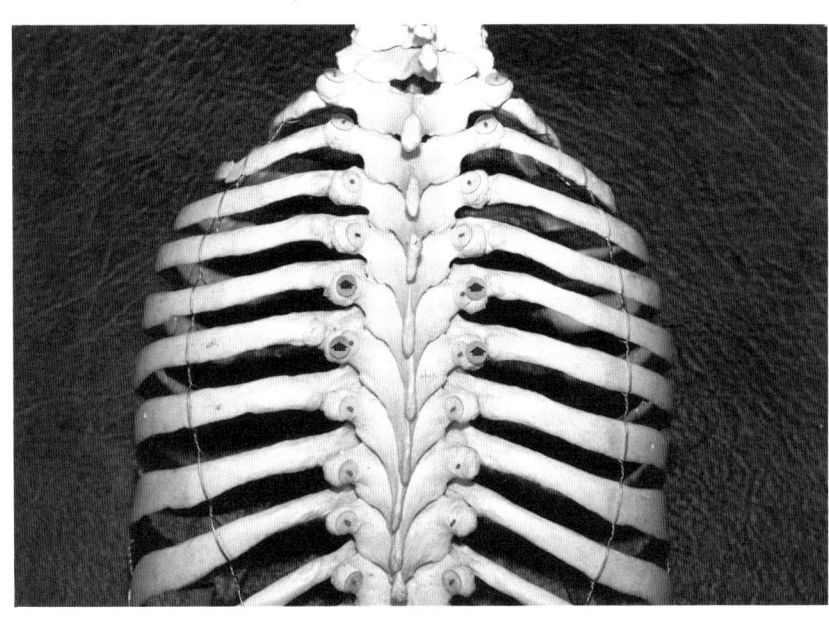
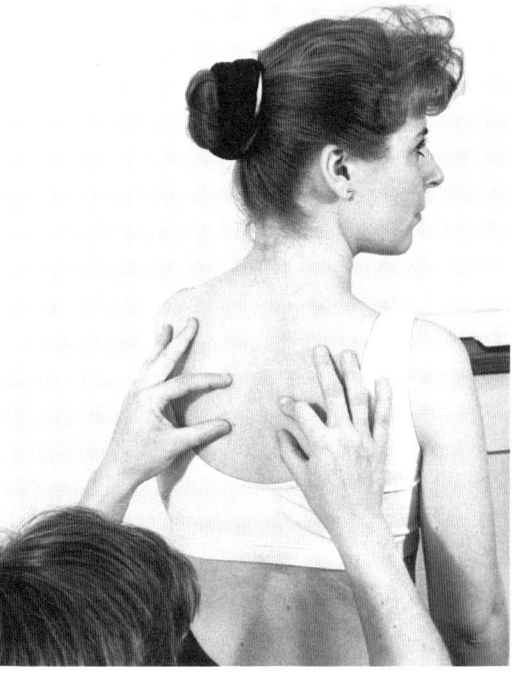

NOTES: _____

_____

_____

_____

_____

_____

_____

ACTIVE MOBILITY TESTS OF OSTEOKINEMATIC FUNCTION — COSTAL

Forward bending

Patient:	Sitting.
Therapist:	Standing behind the patient.
Palpate:	With the thumb of one hand, palpate the rib just lateral to the tubercle and medial to the angle. The index finger of this hand rests along the shaft of the rib. With the thumb of the other hand, palpate the transverse process to which the rib attaches.
Test:	Instruct the patient to forward bend the trunk and note the quantity and direction of relative motion between the vertebra and the rib. The quantity and direction will depend on the relative flexibility between the spinal and costal components. When interpreting the mobility findings, the position of the joint at the beginning of the test should be correlated with the subsequent mobility noted, since alterations in joint mobility may merely be a reflection of an altered starting position.

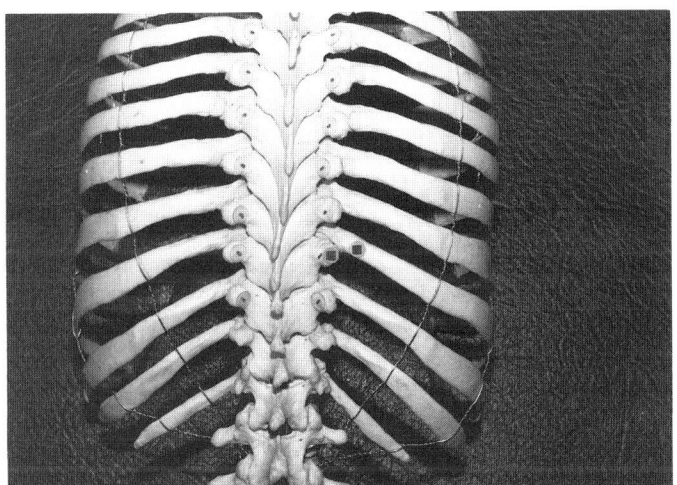
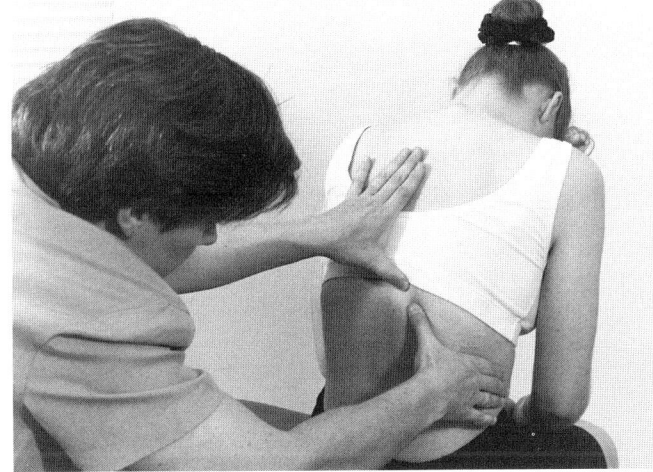

NOTES:

_____

_____

_____

_____

_____

_____

_____

ACTIVE MOBILITY TESTS OF OSTEOKINEMATIC FUNCTION — COSTAL

Backward bending

Patient:	Sitting.
Therapist:	Standing behind the patient.
Palpate:	With the thumb of one hand, palpate the rib just lateral to the tubercle and medial to the angle. The index finger of this hand rests along the shaft of the rib. With the thumb of the other hand, palpate the transverse process to which the rib attaches.
Test:	Instruct the patient to backward bend the trunk and note the quantity and direction of relative motion between the vertebra and the rib. The quantity and direction will depend on the relative flexibility between the spinal and costal components. When interpreting the mobility findings, the position of the joint at the beginning of the test should be correlated with the subsequent mobility noted, since alterations in joint mobility may merely be a reflection of an altered starting position.

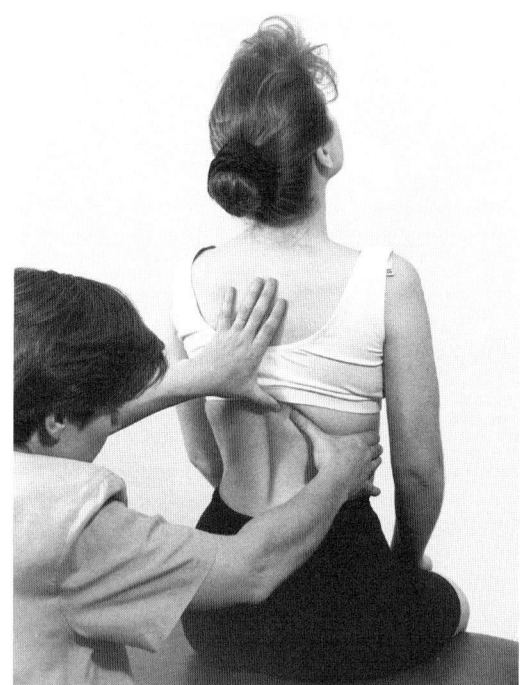

NOTES:

_____

_____

_____

ACTIVE MOBILITY TESTS OF OSTEOKINEMATIC FUNCTION — COSTAL

Lateral bending

Patient:	Sitting.
Therapist:	Standing behind the patient.
Palpate:	With the thumb of one hand, palpate the rib just lateral to the tubercle and medial to the angle. The index finger of this hand rests along the shaft of the rib. With the thumb of the other hand, palpate the transverse process to which the rib attaches.
Test:	Instruct the patient to laterally bend the trunk and note the quantity and direction of relative motion between the vertebra and the rib. When interpreting the mobility findings, the position of the joint at the beginning of the test should be correlated with the subsequent mobility noted since alterations in joint mobility may merely be a reflection of an altered starting position.

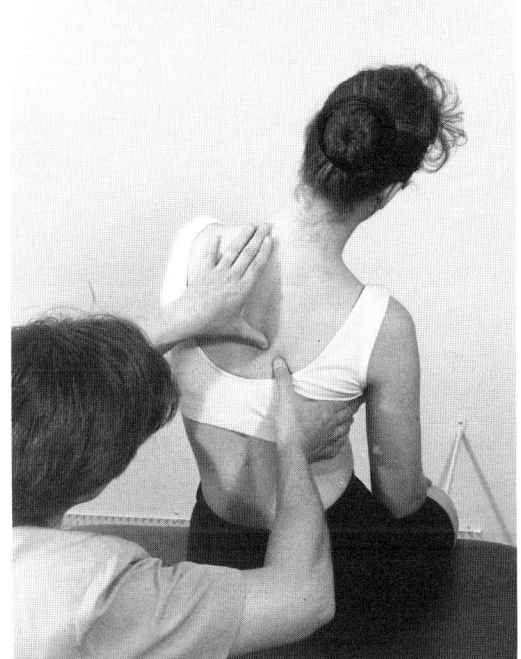

NOTES: _____

_____

_____

_____

_____

ACTIVE MOBILITY TESTS OF OSTEOKINEMATIC FUNCTION — COSTAL

Rotation

Patient: Sitting.

Therapist: Standing behind the patient.

Palpate: With the thumb of one hand, palpate the rib just lateral to the tubercle and medial to the angle. The index finger of this hand rests along the shaft of the rib. With the thumb of the other hand, palpate the transverse process to which the rib attaches.

Test: Instruct the patient to rotate the trunk and note the quantity and direction of relative motion between the vertebra and the rib. When interpreting the mobility findings, the position of the joint at the beginning of the test should be correlated with the subsequent mobility noted since alterations in joint mobility may merely be a reflection of an altered starting position.

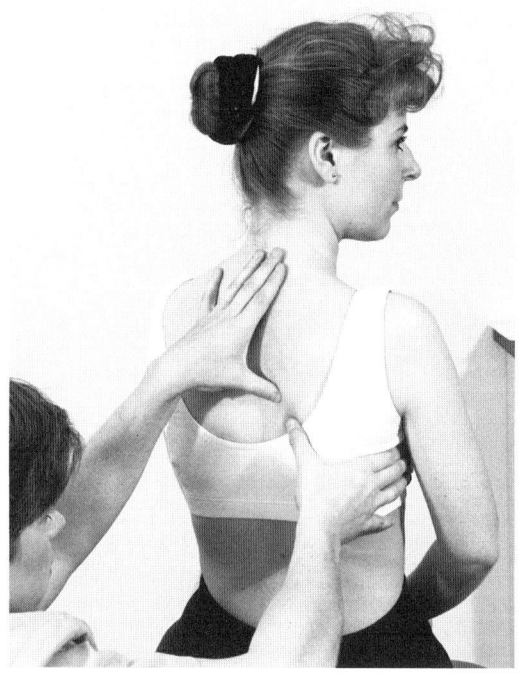

NOTES:

_____

_____

_____

_____

_____

ACTIVE MOBILITY TESTS OF OSTEOKINEMATIC FUNCTION — COSTAL

Respiration

Patient:	Sitting.
Therapist:	Standing behind the patient.
Palpate:	With the thumb of one hand, palpate the rib just lateral to the tubercle and medial to the angle. The index finger of this hand rests along the shaft of the rib. With the thumb of the other hand, palpate the transverse process to which the rib attaches.
Test:	Instruct the patient to take a deep breath in and note the quantity and direction of relative motion between the vertebra and the rib. Instruct the patient to breathe out and note the quantity and direction of relative motion between the vertebra and the rib. When interpreting the mobility findings, the position of the joint at the beginning of the test should be correlated with the subsequent mobility noted since alterations in joint mobility may merely be a reflection of an altered starting position.

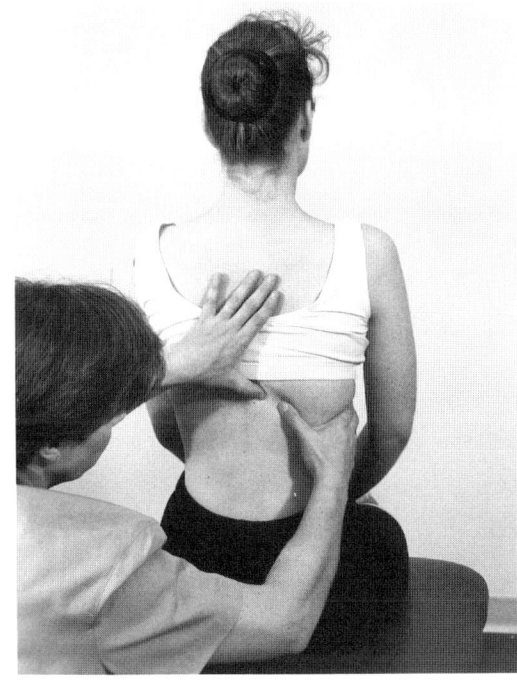

NOTES:

_____

_____

_____

PASSIVE MOBILITY TESTS OF OSTEOKINEMATIC FUNCTION

Flexion/extension/lateral bending/rotation

Patient: Sitting, feet supported, arms crossed to opposite shoulders.
Therapist: Standing at the patient's side.
Palpate: With the index finger of the dorsal hand, palpate the intertransverse space of the segment. For the upper thoracic region, the ventral hand is wound through the patient's crossed arms to rest on the contralateral shoulder. For the lower joints, the ventral hand is placed on the contralateral scapula with the arm resting against the patient's chest. If possible, the ventral hand should be at the level of the cranial vertebra of the joint complex being tested.
Test: Passively flex, extend, laterally bend and rotate the segment and note the quantity, quality, direction of ease and the end feel of motion.

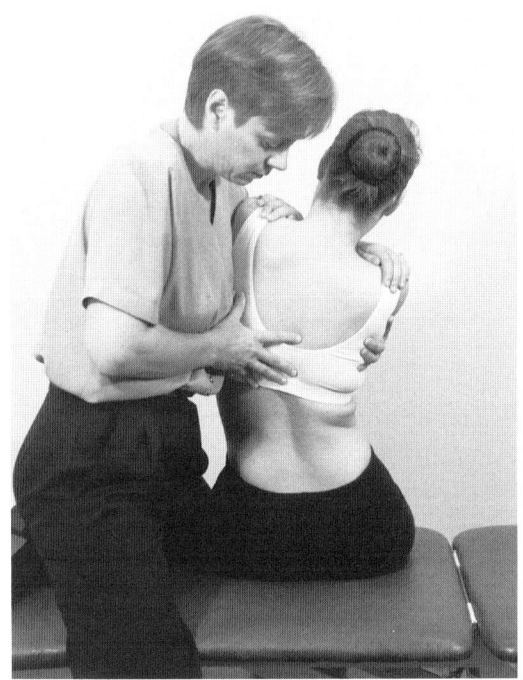

NOTES: _____

_____

_____

_____

_____

PASSIVE MOBILITY TESTS OF ARTHROKINEMATIC FUNCTION — SPINAL

Superoanterior glide – right T4-5 zygapophysial joint

Patient:	Prone.
Therapist:	Standing at the patient's side.
Palpate:	With the left thumb, palpate the inferior aspect of the left transverse process of T5. With the right thumb, palpate the inferior aspect of the right transverse process of T4.
Test:	Fix T5 and apply a force, varying the mediolateral inclination, to produce a superoanterior glide of the right zygapophysial joint at T4-5. Note the quantity, direction of ease and the end feel of motion.

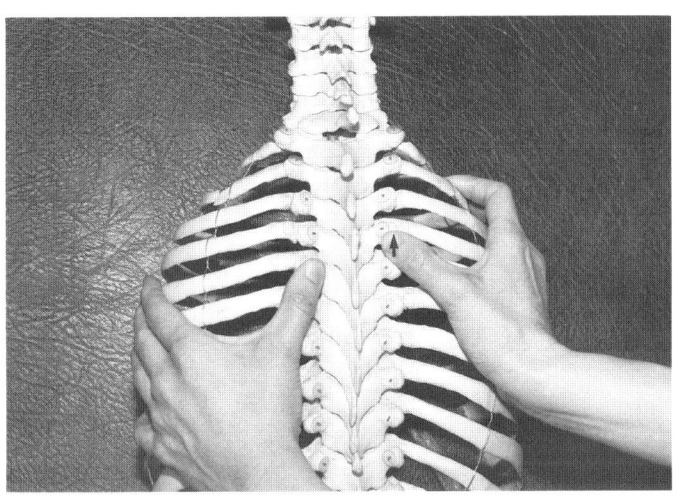
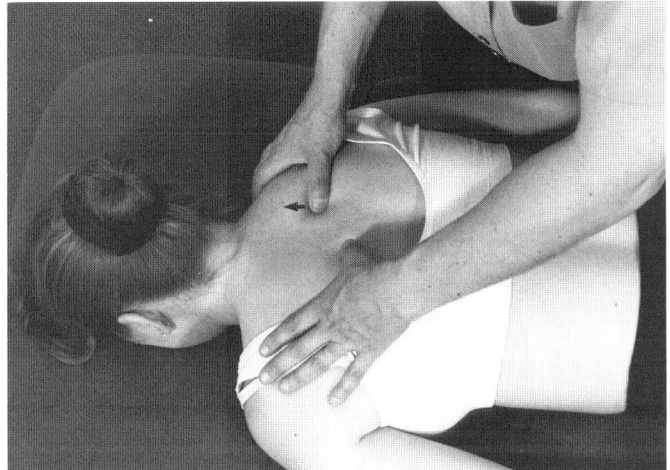

NOTES:

_____

_____

_____

_____

_____

_____

_____

_____

_____

_____

PASSIVE MOBILITY TESTS OF ARTHROKINEMATIC FUNCTION — SPINAL

Inferoposterior glide – right T4-5 zygapophysial joint

Patient: Prone.

Therapist: Standing at the patient's side.

Palpate: With the left thumb, palpate the inferior aspect of the right transverse process of T5. With the right thumb, palpate the superior aspect of the right transverse process of T4.

Test: Fix T5 with an anterosuperior pressure and apply a force to produce an inferior glide of the right zygapophysial joint at T4-5 with the right thumb. Note the quantity, direction of ease and the end feel of motion.

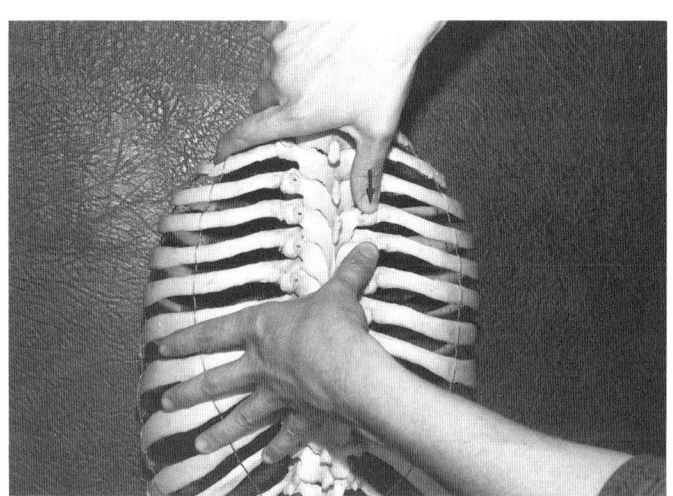 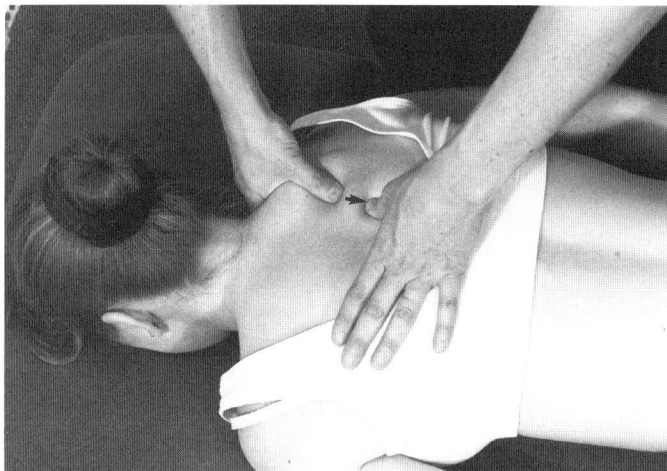

NOTES:

_____

_____

_____

_____

_____

_____

_____

_____

_____

_____

PASSIVE MOBILITY TESTS OF ARTHROKINEMATIC FUNCTION — COSTAL

Inferior glide/posterior roll – right fifth costotransverse joint

Patient:	Prone.
Therapist:	Standing at the patient's side.
Palpate:	With the left thumb, palpate the inferior aspect of the right transverse process of T5. With the right thumb, palpate the superior aspect of the right fifth rib just lateral to the tubercle.
Test:	Fix T5 and apply a force to produce an inferior glide of the right fifth costotransverse joint. Allow the conjunct posterior roll to occur. Note the quantity, direction of ease and the end feel of motion.
Addendum:	Between T7 and T10 the orientation of the costotransverse joint changes and the direction of the glide is anterolateroinferior. The position of the right hand is modified such that the index finger of the right hand lies along the shaft of the rib.

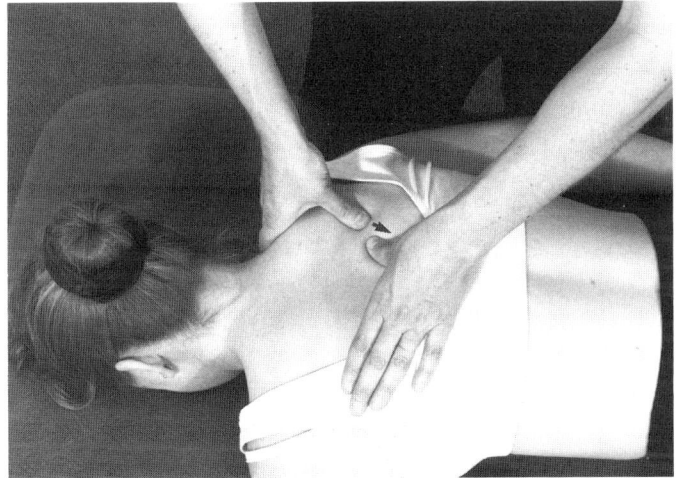
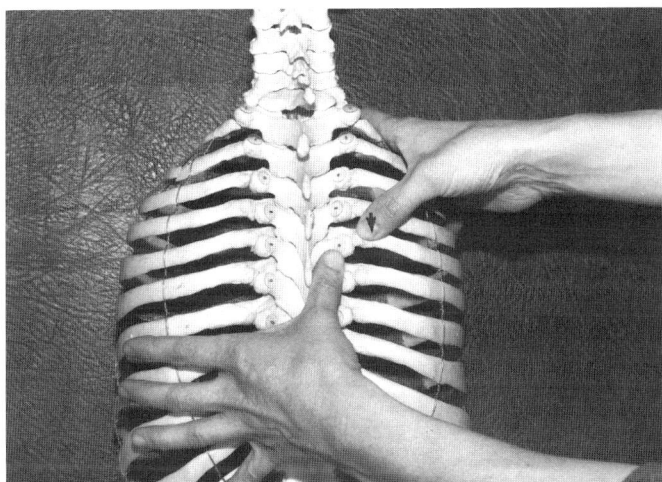
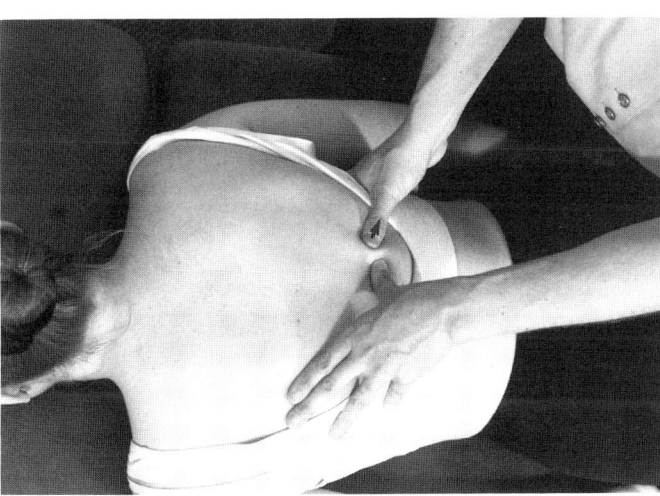
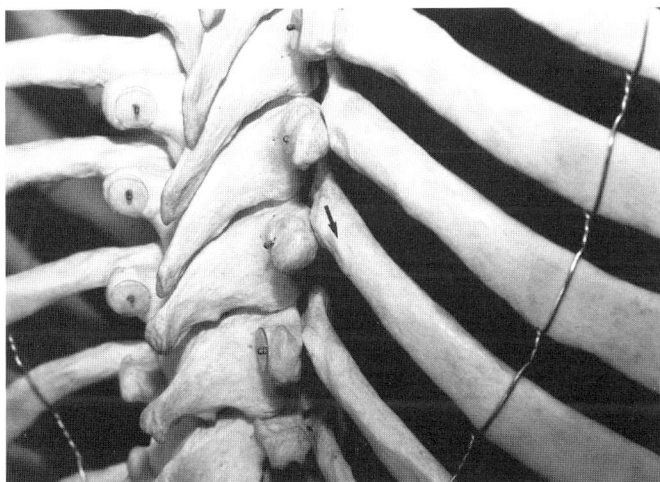

PASSIVE MOBILITY TESTS OF ARTHROKINEMATIC FUNCTION — COSTAL

Superior glide/anterior roll – right fifth costotransverse joint

Patient: Prone.

Therapist: Standing at the patient's side.

Palpate: With the right thumb, palpate the superior aspect of the right transverse process of T5. With the left thumb, palpate the inferior aspect of the right fifth rib just lateral to the tubercle.

Test: Fix T5 and apply a force to produce a superior glide of the right fifth costotransverse joint. Allow the conjunct anterior roll to occur. Note the quantity, direction of ease and the end feel of motion.

Addendum: Between T7 and T10 the orientation of the costotransverse joint changes and the direction of the glide is posteromediosuperior. The position of the right hand is modified such that the index finger of the right hand lies along the shaft of the rib. The right hand fixes the rib and the left hand glides the transverse process anterolateroinferior thus producing a posteromediosuperior glide at the costotransverse joint.

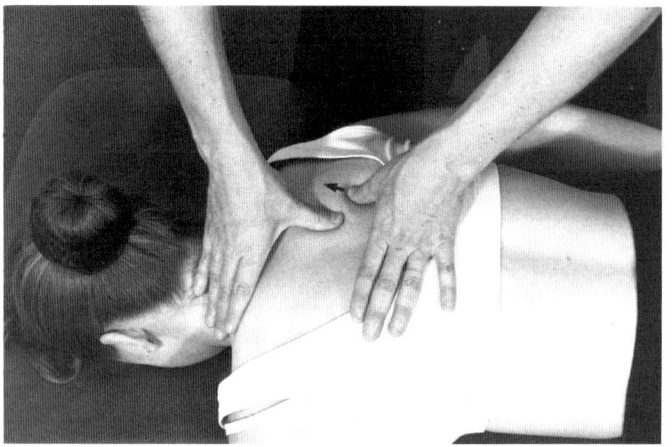
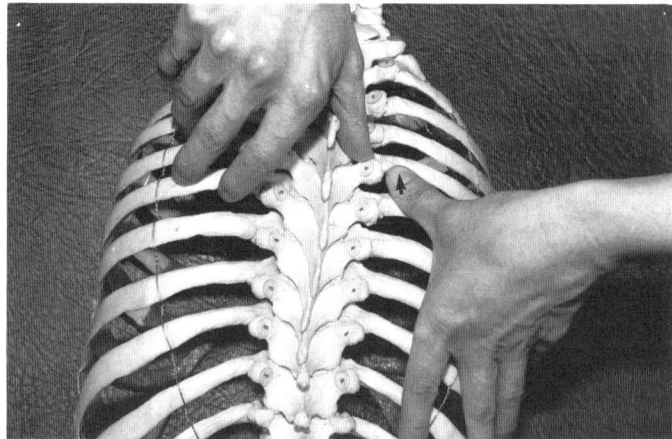
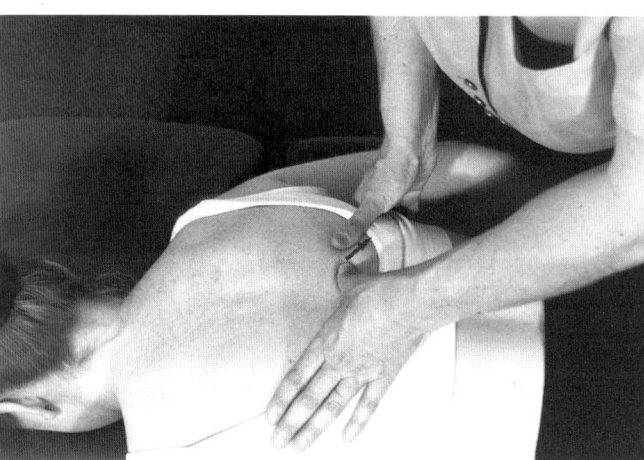
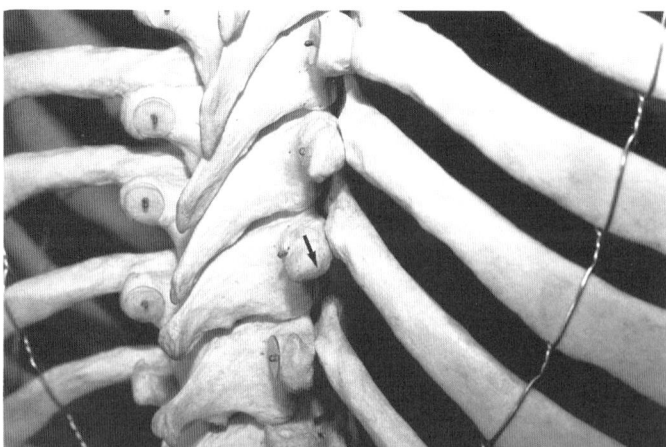

PASSIVE MOBILITY TESTS OF ARTHROKINEMATIC FUNCTION – RING COMPLEX

Right lateral glide – T5, left and right sixth ribs relative to T6

Patient: Sitting, arms crossed to opposite shoulders.
Therapist: Standing beside the patient.
Palpate: With the right hand/arm palpate the thorax such that the fifth finger of the right hand lies along the left sixth rib. With the left hand, fix the transverse processes of T6.
Test: Fix T6 and apply a PURE right horizontal translation force to the thorax through the left sixth rib. This will translate the sixth ribs and T5 to the right relative to T6. Note the quantity of motion and in particular the end feel of motion.

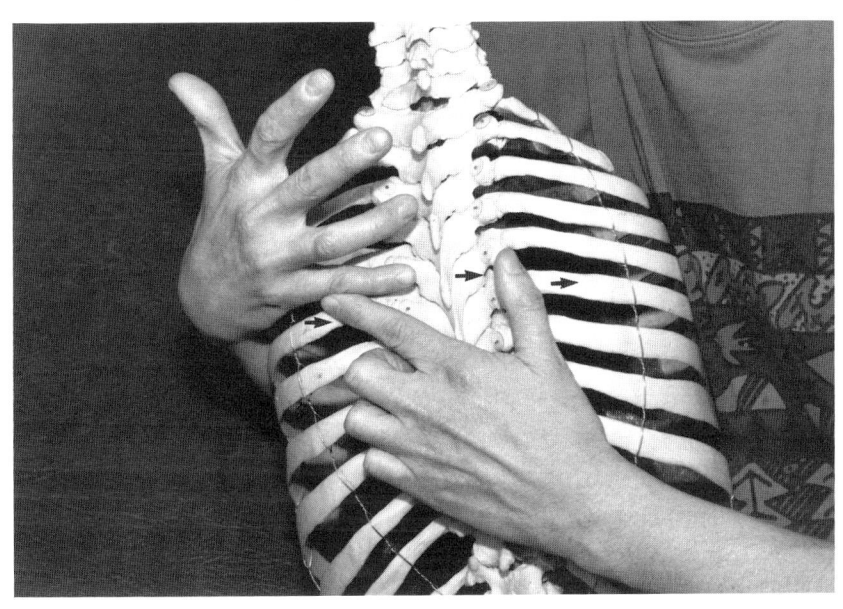 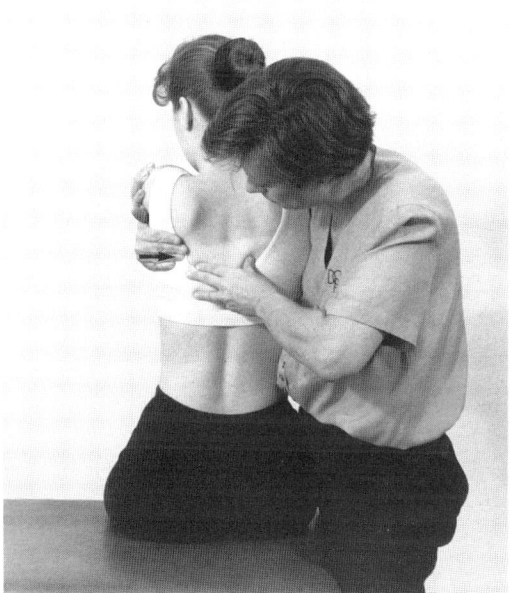

NOTES:

_____

_____

_____

_____

_____

_____

_____

_____

THORACIC
REGION

PASSIVE STABILITY TESTS OF ARTHROKINETIC FUNCTION – SPINAL

Vertical (traction/compression)

Patient: Sitting, feet supported, with the arms crossed to opposite shoulders such that the arm closest to the chest grasps the scapula.
Therapist: Standing behind the patient.
Palpate: Traction – With fingers interlaced, grasp the patient's flexed elbow closest to the chest.
Compression – With both hands, palpate the top of the patient's shoulders.
Test: Traction vertically in a cranial direction through the patient's crossed arms. Compress vertically in a caudal direction through the top of the patient's shoulders. The force is sustained for 20 seconds. Note the reproduction of any symptoms.

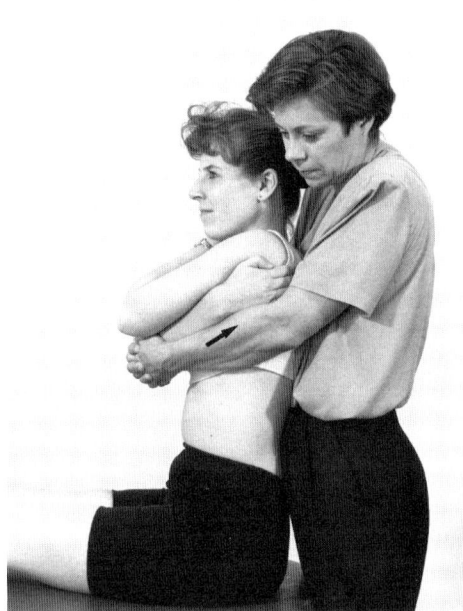 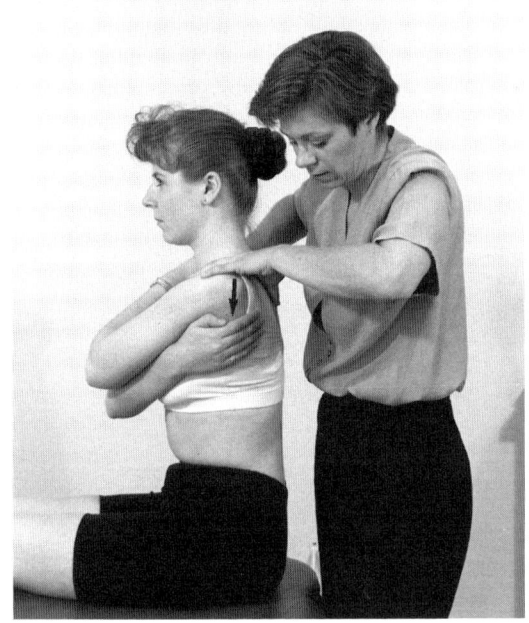

NOTES:

_____

_____

_____

_____

_____

PASSIVE STABILITY TESTS OF ARTHROKINETIC FUNCTION — SPINAL

Anterior translation

Patient:	Prone.
Therapist:	Standing at the patient's side.
Palpate:	With one hand, palpate the transverse processes of the cranial vertebra. With the other hand, palpate the transverse processes of the caudal vertebra.
Test:	Fix the caudal vertebra and apply a posteroanterior force to the cranial vertebra in a PURE horizontal plane. Sustain the force until the end feel is perceived. Note the quantity and end feel of motion as well as the reproduction of any symptoms.
Addendum:	The findings from this test should be correlated with those of the posterior translation test to determine the segmental level of instability.

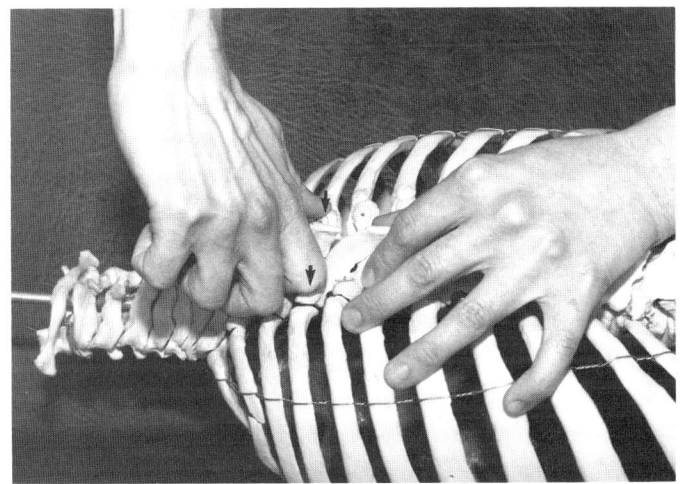 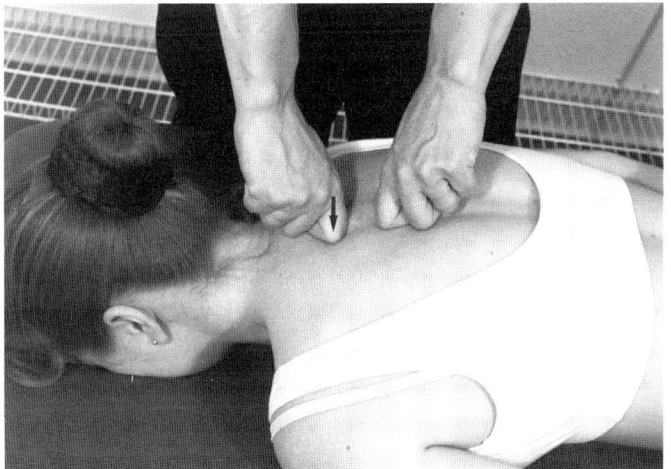

NOTES:

_____

_____

_____

_____

_____

_____

_____

_____

PASSIVE STABILITY TESTS OF ARTHROKINETIC FUNCTION — SPINAL

Posterior translation

Patient:	Sitting, arms crossed to opposite shoulders.
Therapist:	Standing at the patient's side.
Palpate:	With the dorsal hand, palpate the transverse processes of the caudal vertebra. With the ventral hand, palpate the thorax over the patient's crossed arms at the level of the cranial vertebra.
Test:	Fix the caudal vertebra and apply an anteroposterior force to the cranial vertebra in a PURE horizontal plane. Sustain the force until the end feel is perceived. Note the quantity and end feel of motion as well as the reproduction of any symptoms.
Addendum:	The findings from this test should be correlated with those of the anterior translation test to determine the segmental level of instability.

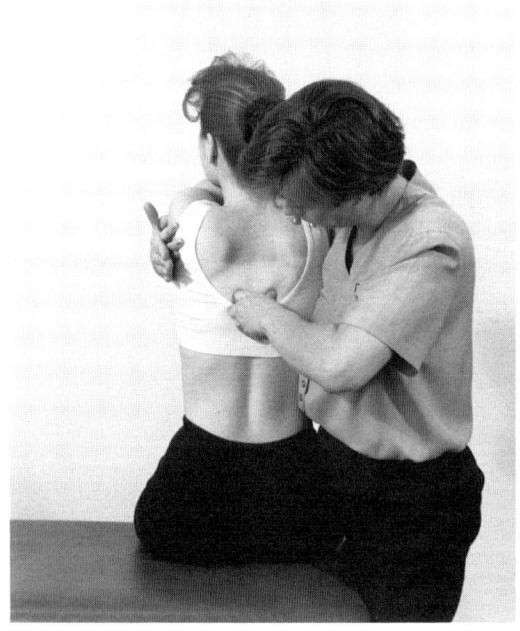

NOTES:

_____

_____

_____

_____

_____

PASSIVE STABILITY TESTS OF ARTHROKINETIC FUNCTION — SPINAL

Rotation

Patient:	Prone.
Therapist:	Standing at the patient's side.
Palpate:	With one hand, palpate the transverse process of the cranial vertebra. With the other hand, palpate the contralateral transverse process of the caudal vertebra.
Test:	Fix the caudal vertebra and apply a posteroanterior force unilaterally to the cranial vertebra in a PURE horizontal plane. Sustain the force until the end feel is perceived. Note the quantity and end feel of motion as well as the reproduction of any symptoms.

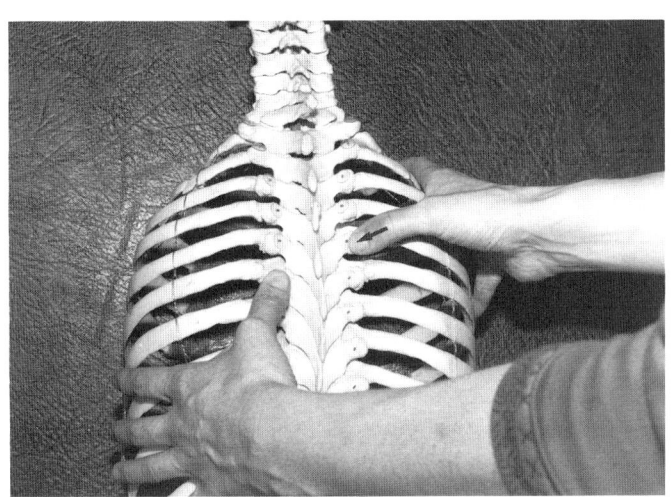 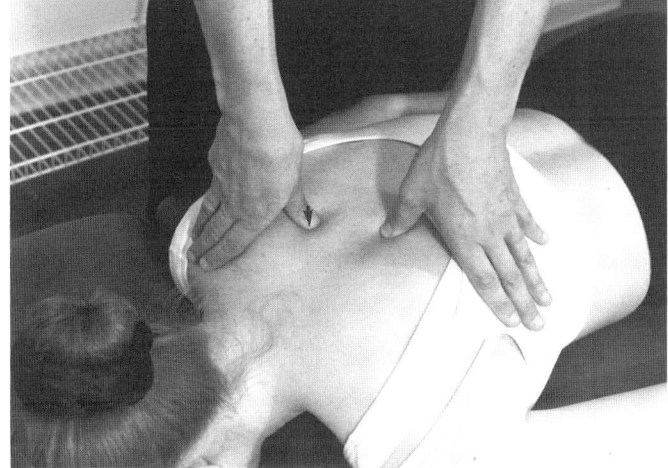

NOTES:

_____

_____

_____

_____

_____

_____

_____

_____

_____

_____

PASSIVE STABILITY TESTS OF ARTHROKINETIC FUNCTION – COSTAL

Posterior costal joints – anterior translation

Patient: Prone.

Therapist: Standing at the patient's side.

Palpate: With one hand, palpate the rib just lateral to the tubercle. With the other hand, palpate the contralateral transverse processes of the two thoracic vertebra to which the rib attaches.

Test: Fix the thoracic vertebrae and apply a posteroanterior force to the rib in a PURE horizontal plane. Sustain the force until the end feel is perceived. Note the quantity and end feel of motion as well as the reproduction any symptoms.

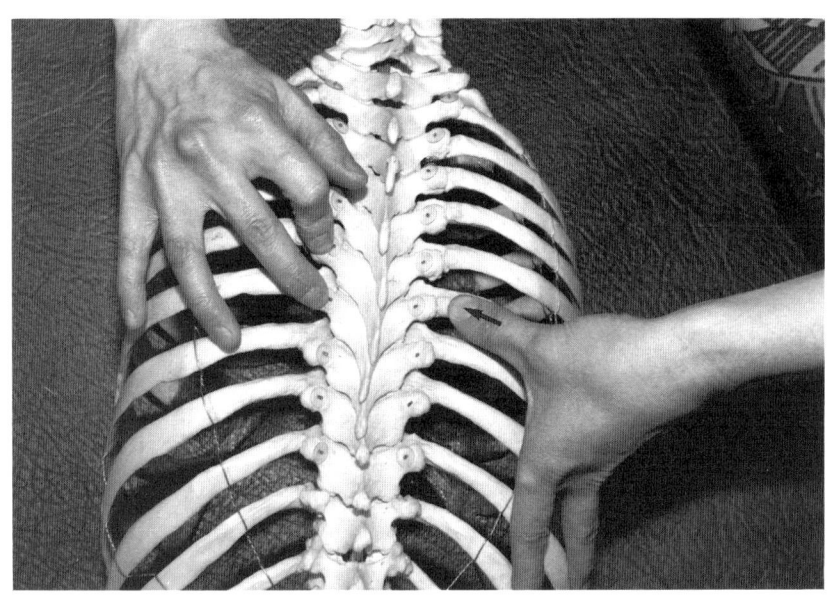
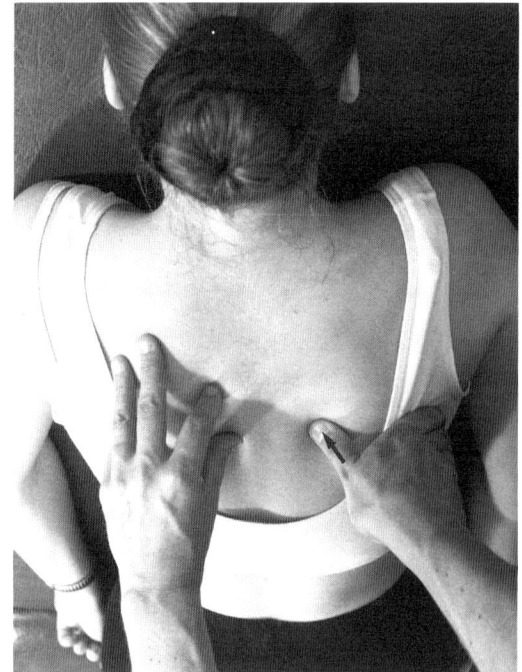

NOTES: _____

_____

_____

_____

_____

_____

_____

PASSIVE STABILITY TESTS OF ARTHROKINETIC FUNCTION – COSTAL

Posterior costal joints – inferior translation

Patient: Prone.

Therapist: Standing at the patient's head facing the shoulders.

Palpate: With one hand, palpate the superior aspect of the rib just lateral to the tubercle. With the other hand, palpate the contralateral transverse process of the thoracic vertebra at the same level as the rib. With the same hand, palpate the ipsilateral transverse process of the thoracic vertebra of the level above the rib.

Test: Fix the thoracic vertebrae and apply a superoinferior force to the rib. Sustain the force until the end feel is perceived. Note the quantity and end feel of motion as well as the reproduction of any symptoms.

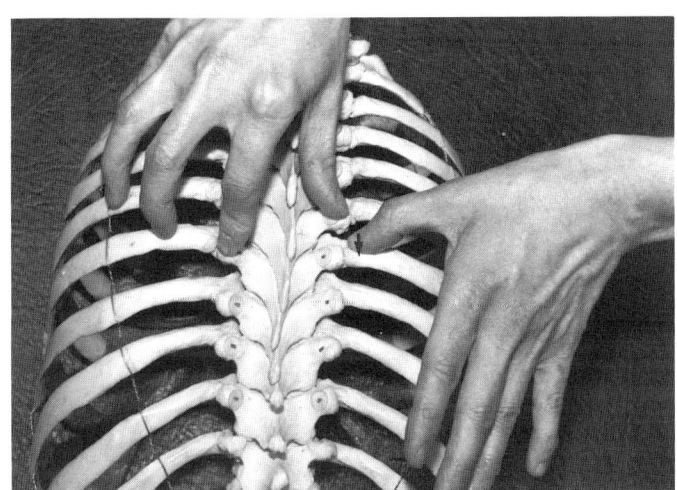 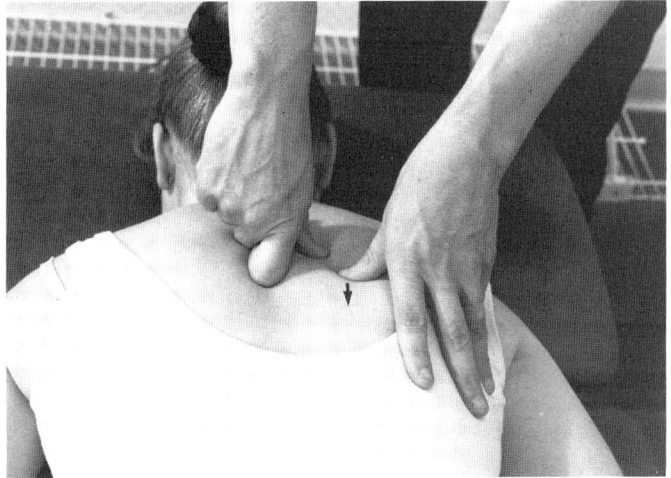

NOTES:

_____

_____

_____

_____

_____

_____

_____

_____

PASSIVE STABILITY TESTS OF ARTHROKINETIC FUNCTION – COSTAL

Anterior costal joints – anteroposterior translation

Patient: Supine.
Therapist: Standing at the patient's side.
Palpate: With one thumb, palpate the sternum/costal cartilage. With the other thumb, palpate the anterior aspect of the costal cartilage/rib.
Test: Apply an anteroposterior force to the:
a) sternum (sternocostal junction)
b) sternal end of the costal cartilage (sternocostal junction)
c) costal end of the costal cartilage (costochondral junction)
d) cartilagenous end of the rib (costochondral junction)
Sustain the force until the end feel is perceived. Note the quantity of motion, the reproduction of any symptoms and the end feel of motion.

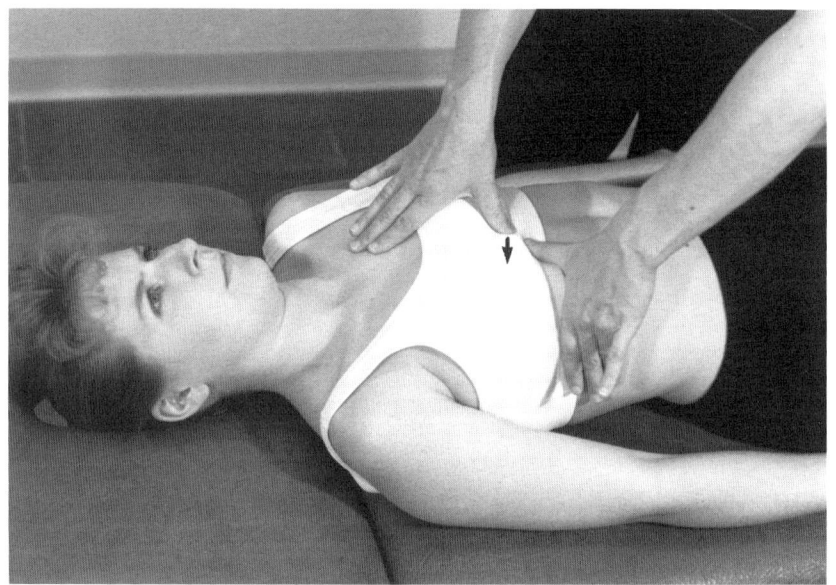

NOTES: _____
_____
_____
_____
_____
_____
_____

PASSIVE STABILITY TESTS OF ARTHROKINETIC FUNCTION – COSTAL

Anterior costal joints – superoinferior translation

Patient:	Supine.
Therapist:	Standing at the patient's side.
Palpate:	With one thumb, palpate the sternum/costal cartilage. With the other thumb, palpate the superior or inferior aspect of the costal cartilage or rib.
Test:	Apply a superoinferior force to the: **a)** sternum (sternocostal junction) **b)** sternal end of the costal cartilage (sternocostal junction) (arrow) **c)** costal end of the costal cartilage (costochondral junction) **d)** cartilagenous end of the rib (costochondral junction) Sustain the force until the end feel is perceived. Note the quantity of motion, the reproduction of any symptoms and the end feel of motion.

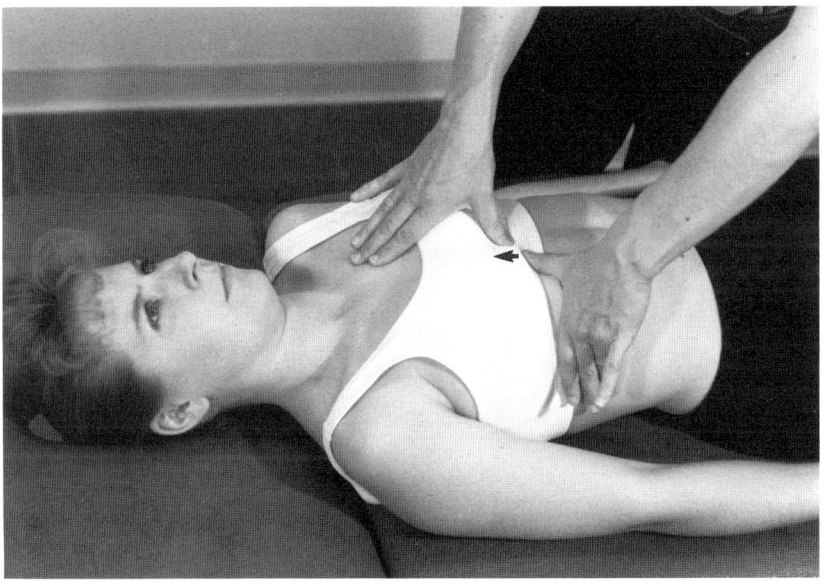

NOTES:

_____

_____

_____

_____

_____

_____

PASSIVE STABILITY TESTS OF ARTHROKINETIC FUNCTION — RING COMPLEX

Right horizontal translation of T5-6

Patient:	Sitting, arms crossed to opposite shoulders.
Therapist:	Standing beside the patient.
Palpate:	With the right hand/arm, palpate the thorax such that the fifth finger of the right hand lies along the left fifth rib. With the left hand, fix T6 by compressing the sixth ribs centrally towards their costovertebral joints.
Test:	Fix T6 and apply a PURE right horizontal translation force to the thorax through the left fifth rib. The primary structure being tested is the intervertebral disc. Sustain the force until the end feel is perceived. Note the quantity of motion and in particular the end feel of motion.

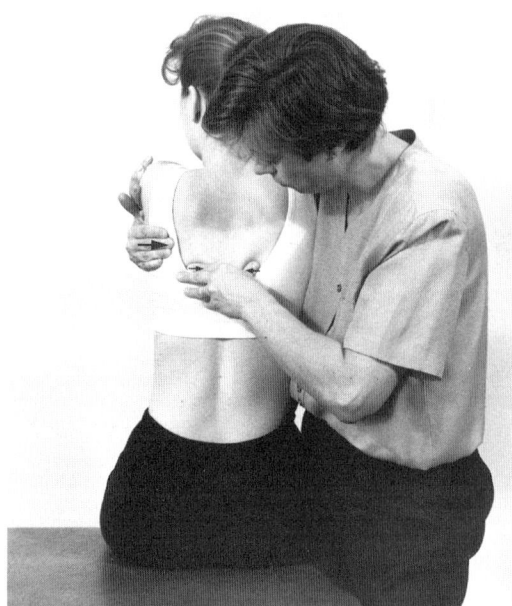

NOTES:

_____

_____

_____

_____

_____

_____

_____

MOBILIZATION TECHNIQUES — SPINAL

Specific traction

Patient: Side lying, arms crossed to opposite shoulders.

Therapist: Standing facing the patient.

Palpate: With the tubercle of the scaphoid bone and the PIP of the long finger, palpate the transverse processes of the caudal vertebra. The other hand/arm lies across the patient's crossed arms to control the thorax.

Localization: To isolate the neutral position, flex the joint to the motion barrier and then return the joint to neutral with the hand controlling the thorax. Maintain this neutral position and roll the patient supine, only until sufficient contact is made between the dorsal hand and the table.

Mobilization: Fix the caudal vertebra and apply a grade 1 to 5 traction force through the thorax.

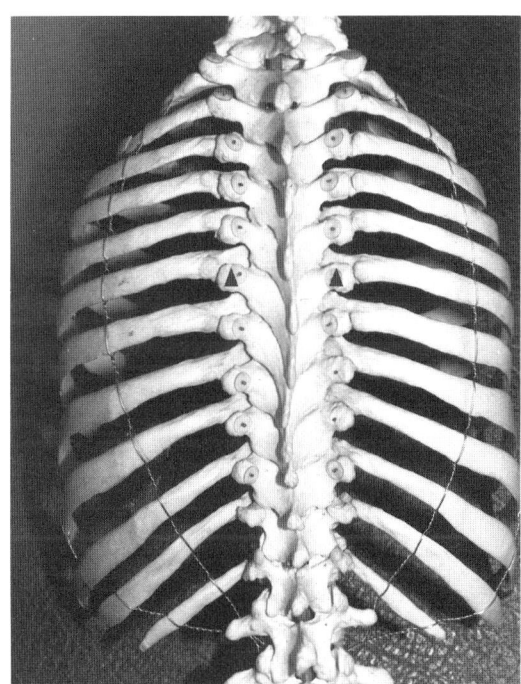
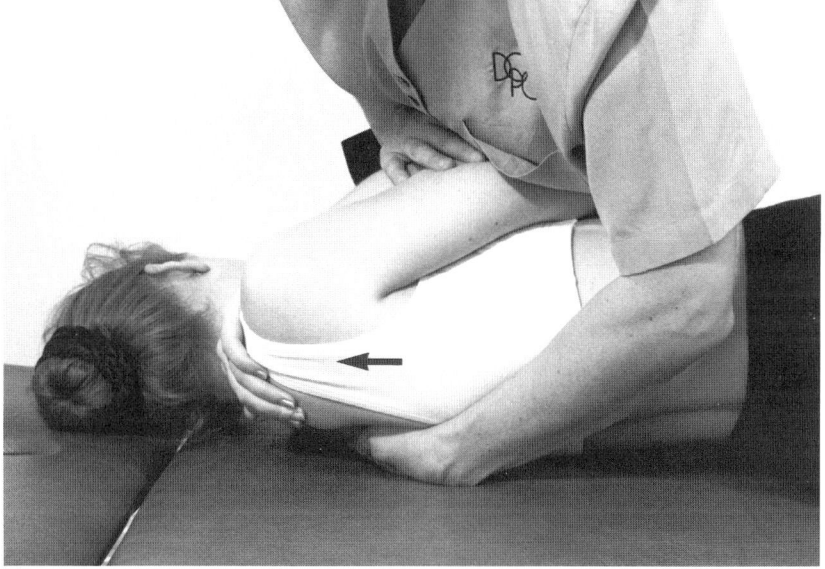

NOTES:

_____

_____

_____

_____

_____

MOBILIZATION TECHNIQUES — SPINAL

Regional traction

Patient: Sitting, arms crossed to opposite shoulders.

Therapist: Standing behind the patient.

Palpate: Place a small rolled towel against the spinous process of the caudal vertebra. Fix the towel against the therapist's sternum. With fingers interlaced, palpate the patient's flexed elbow closest to their chest. Grip the thorax with the inner arms.

Localization: To isolate the neutral position, flex and extend the joint to the motion barrier and then return the joint to neutral.

Mobilization: Maintain this neutral position and apply a grade 2 to 5 traction force by rocking the patient backwards and lifting the thorax posterosuperiorly through the patient's elbow.

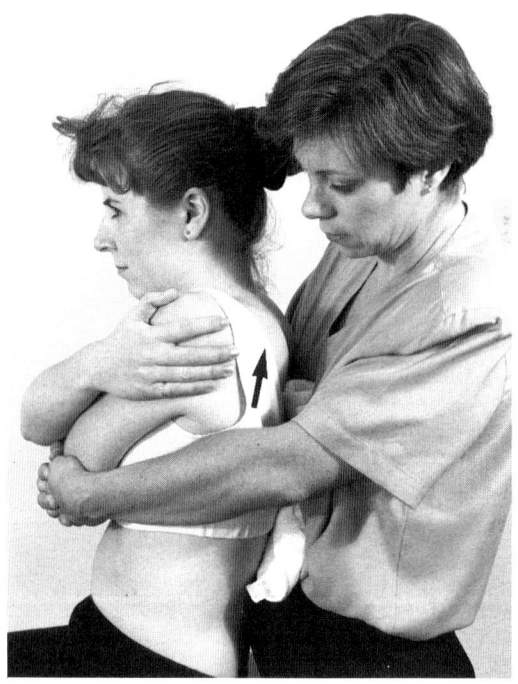

NOTES:

_____

_____

_____

_____

_____

MOBILIZATION TECHNIQUES – SPINAL

Restriction of flexion/right lateral bending/rotation (superoanteromedial glide) – left T5-6 zygapophysial joint

Supine

Patient: Side lying, arms crossed to opposite shoulders.

Therapist: Standing facing the patient.

Palpate: With the tubercle of the right scaphoid bone and the flexed PIP joint of the right long finger, palpate the left transverse process of T6 and the right transverse process of T5. The other arm/hand lies across the patient's crossed arms to control the thorax.

Localization: Flex the joint to the motion barrier with the hand controlling the thorax. Maintain this flexion and roll the patient supine, only until sufficient contact is made between the dorsal hand and the table.

Mobilization: **Passive** – Apply a grade 3 to 5 right lateral bending force (arrow) through the thorax to produce a superoanteromedial glide of the left zygapophysial joint at T5-6.

Active – From the motion barrier, instruct the patient to gently elevate their arms. The isometric contraction is held for up to 5 seconds and followed by a period of complete relaxation. The joint is then passively taken to the new motion barrier. This technique is repeated 3 times and followed by a re-evaluation of osteokinematic, arthrokinematic and arthrokinetic function.

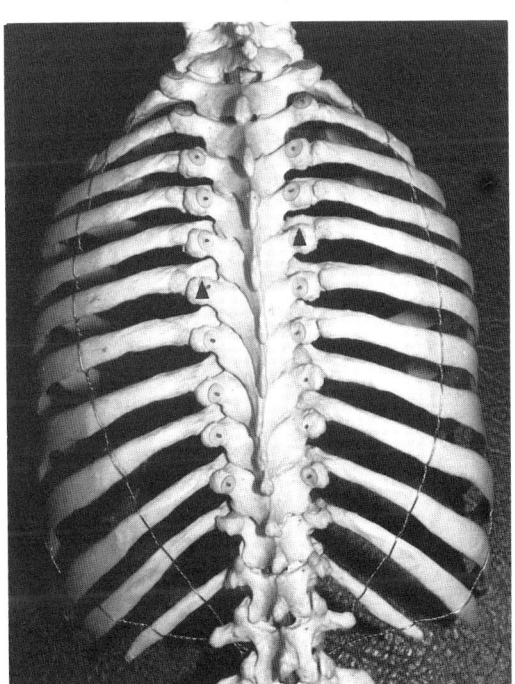

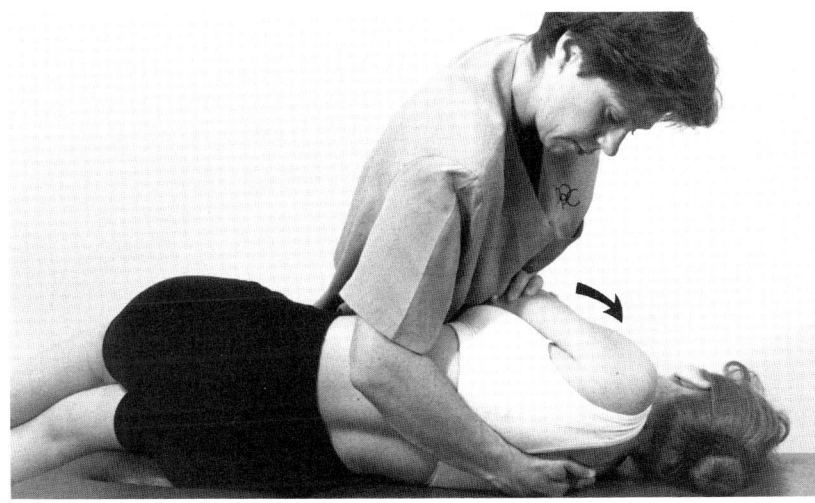

MOBILIZATION TECHNIQUES — SPINAL

Restriction of flexion/right lateral bending/rotation – T5-6

Sitting

Patient: Sitting, arms crossed to opposite shoulders.

Therapist: Standing at the patient's side.

Palpate: With the dorsal hand, palpate the intertransverse space. The other hand/arm rests on the contralateral shoulder to control the thorax.

Localization: The motion barrier is localized with flexion and right lateral bending/rotation.

Mobilization: **Active** – From this position, the patient is instructed to hold still while the therapist applies a resistance to the trunk. The direction of resistance is that which facilitates flexion/right lateral bending/rotation. The isometric contraction is held for up to 5 seconds and followed by a period of complete relaxation. The joint is then passively taken to the new motion barrier. This technique is repeated 3 times and followed by a re-evaluation of osteokinematic, arthrokinematic and arthrokinetic function.

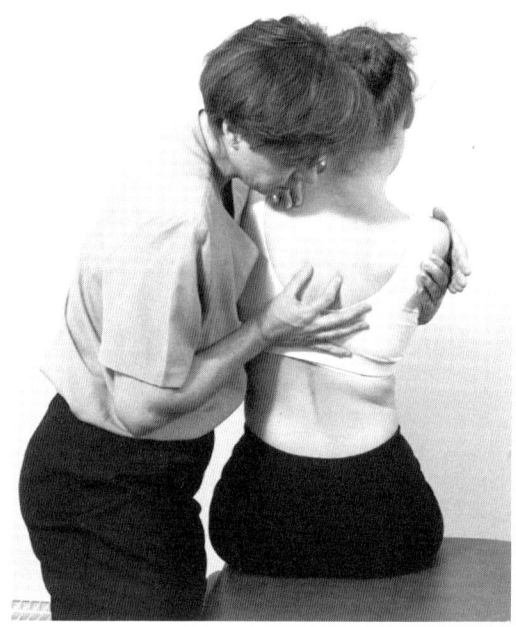

NOTES:

_____

_____

_____

MOBILIZATION TECHNIQUES — SPINAL

Restriction of extension/left lateral bending/rotation (inferoposteromedial glide) – left T5-6 zygapophysial joint

Supine

Patient: Side lying, arms crossed to opposite shoulders.

Therapist: Standing facing the patient.

Palpate: With the tubercle of the right scaphoid bone and the flexed PIP joint of the right long finger, palpate the left transverse process of T6 and the right transverse process of T5. The other arm/hand lies across the patient's crossed arms to control the thorax.

Localization: Extend the joint to the motion barrier with the hand controlling the thorax. Maintain this extension and roll the patient supine, only until sufficient contact is made between the dorsal hand and the table. The left hand is then placed on the superior aspect of the patient's left shoulder.

Mobilization: **Passive** – Apply a grade 2 to 5 left lateral bending force (coupled with a slight dorsal glide) (arrow) through the thorax to produce a grade 2 to 5 inferoposteromedial glide of the left zygapophysial joint at T5-6.

Active – From the motion barrier, instruct the patient to gently elevate their arms. The isometric contraction is held for up to 5 seconds and followed by a period of complete relaxation. The joint is then passively taken to the new motion barrier. This technique is repeated 3 times and followed by re-evaluation of osteokinematic, arthrokinematic and arthrokinetic function.

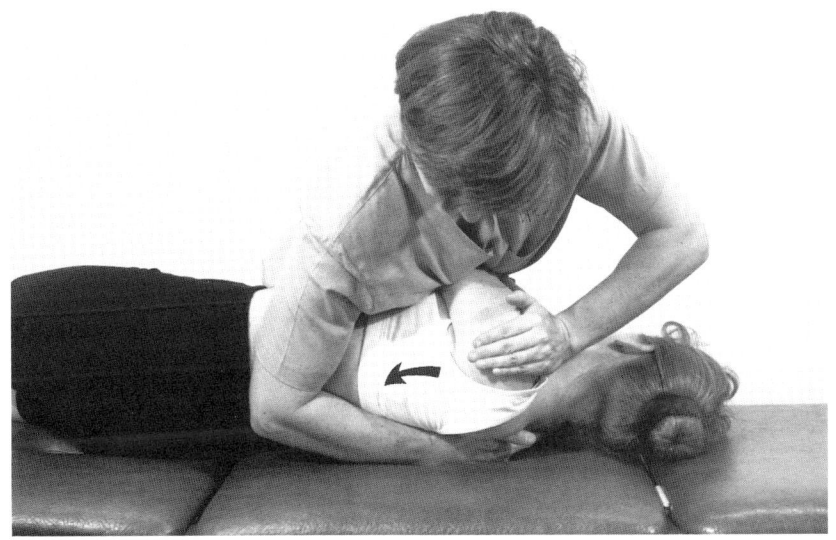

MOBILIZATION TECHNIQUES – SPINAL

Restriction of extension/left lateral bending/rotation – T5-6

Sitting
Patient: Sitting, arms crossed to opposite shoulders.
Therapist: Standing at the patient's side.
Palpate: With the dorsal hand, palpate the intertransverse space. The other hand/arm rests on the contralateral shoulder to control the thorax.
Localization: The motion barrier is localized with extension and left lateral bending/rotation.
Mobilization: **Active** – From this position, the patient is instructed to hold still while the therapist applies a resistance to the trunk. The direction of resistance is that which facilitates extension/left lateral bending/rotation. The isometric contraction is held for up to 5 seconds and followed by a period of complete relaxation. The joint is then passively taken to the new motion barrier. This technique is repeated 3 times and followed by a re-evaluation of osteokinematic, arthrokinematic and arthrokinetic function.

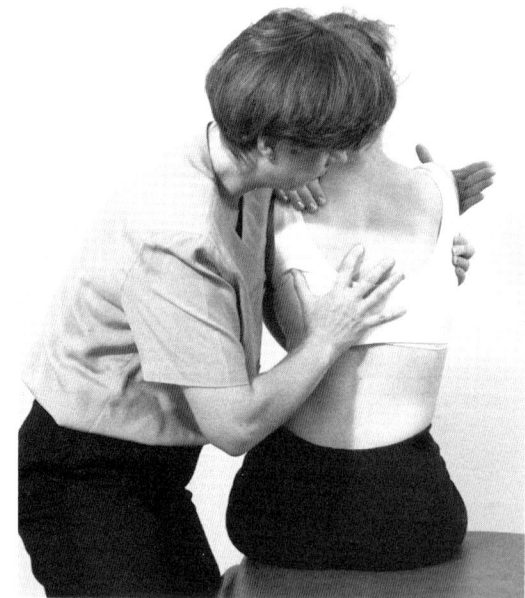

NOTES:

_____

_____

_____

MOBILIZATION TECHNIQUES — COSTAL

Restriction of posterior rotation – right fifth rib

Patient: Sitting, arms crossed to opposite shoulders.

Therapist: Standing at the patient's side.

Palpate: With the thumb and index finger of the dorsal hand, palpate the right fifth rib. The other hand/arm rests on the contralateral shoulder to control the thorax.

Localization: The motion barrier is localized with left lateral bending and right rotation.

Mobilization: **Active** – From this position, the patient is instructed to hold still while the therapist applies a resistance to the trunk. The direction of resistance is that which facilitates posterior rotation of the rib. The isometric contraction is held for up to 5 seconds and followed by a period of complete relaxation. The joint is then passively taken to the new motion barrier. This technique is repeated 3 times and followed by a re-evaluation of osteokinematic, arthrokinematic and arthrokinetic function.

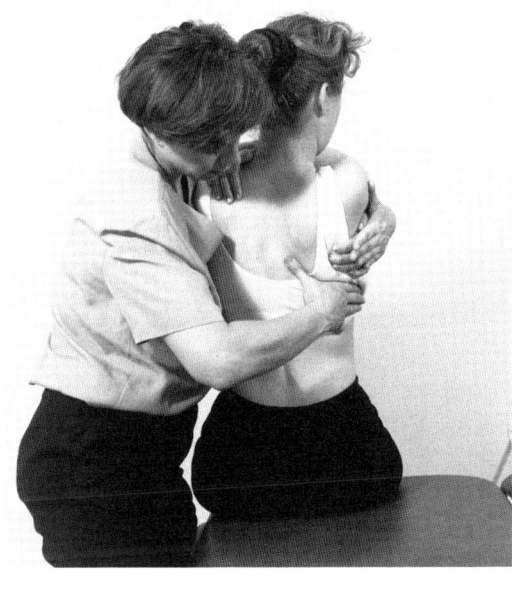

NOTES:

_____

_____

_____

_____

MOBILIZATION TECHNIQUES – COSTAL

Restriction of anterior rotation – right fifth rib

Patient: Sitting, arms crossed to opposite shoulders.

Therapist: Standing at the patient's side.

Palpate: With the thumb and index finger of the dorsal hand, palpate the right fifth rib. The other hand/arm rests on the contralateral shoulder to control the thorax.

Localization: The motion barrier is localized with right lateral bending and left rotation.

Mobilization: **Active** – From this position, the patient is instructed to hold still while the therapist applies a resistance to the trunk. The direction of resistance is that which facilitates anterior rotation of the rib. The isometric contraction is held for up to 5 seconds and followed by a period of complete relaxation. The joint is then passively taken to the new motion barrier. This technique is repeated 3 times and followed by a re-evaluation of osteokinematic, arthrokinematic and arthrokinetic function.

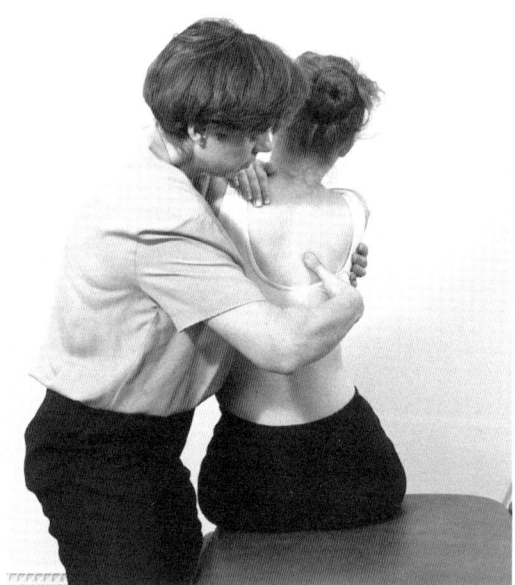

NOTES:

_____

_____

_____

_____

MANIPULATION TECHNIQUES – COSTAL

Subluxed costotransverse joint – ribs 2 - 9 (10)

Patient: Side lying, arms crossed to opposite shoulders.
Therapist: Standing at the patient's side.
Localization: Palpate the rib just lateral to the tubercle with the proximal phalanx of the thumb. The other hand/arm supports the patient's thorax. Maintain this contact and roll the patient supine, only until sufficient contact is made between the dorsal hand and the table.
Mobilization: Continue to axially rotate the thorax against the fixed rib. This is a grade 5 technique and minimal force is required to reduce the subluxation.

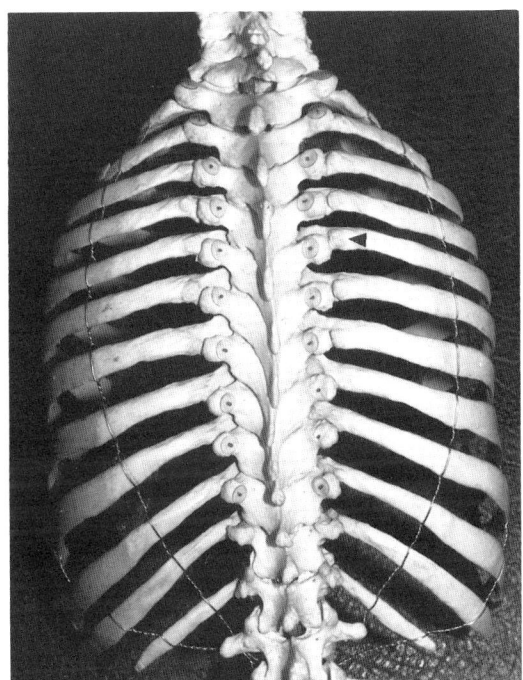
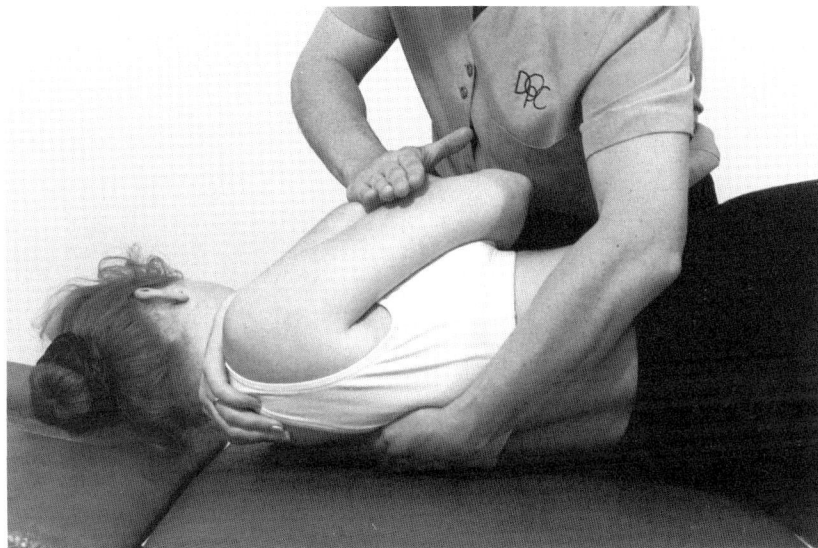

NOTES:

_____

_____

_____

_____

_____

_____

_____

MANIPULATION TECHNIQUES – COSTAL

Subluxed costotransverse joint – right twelfth rib

Patient: Left side lying, hips and knees slightly flexed.

Therapist: Standing facing the patient.

Localization: Palpate the T12 - L1 interspinous space with one hand and rotate the thoracolumbar spine until full right rotation of T12 - L1 is achieved. Palpate the L1 - 2 interspinous space and flex the patient's uppermost hip and knee until full flexion of L1 - 2 is achieved. The foot of the upper leg rests against the popliteal fossa of the lower leg. Palpate the right side of the spinous process of T12 with one hand. With the thumb and index finger of the other hand, palpate and fix the right twelfth rib.

Mobilization: Axially rotate T12 away from the fixed rib with a high velocity, low amplitude thrust. This is a grade 5 technique.

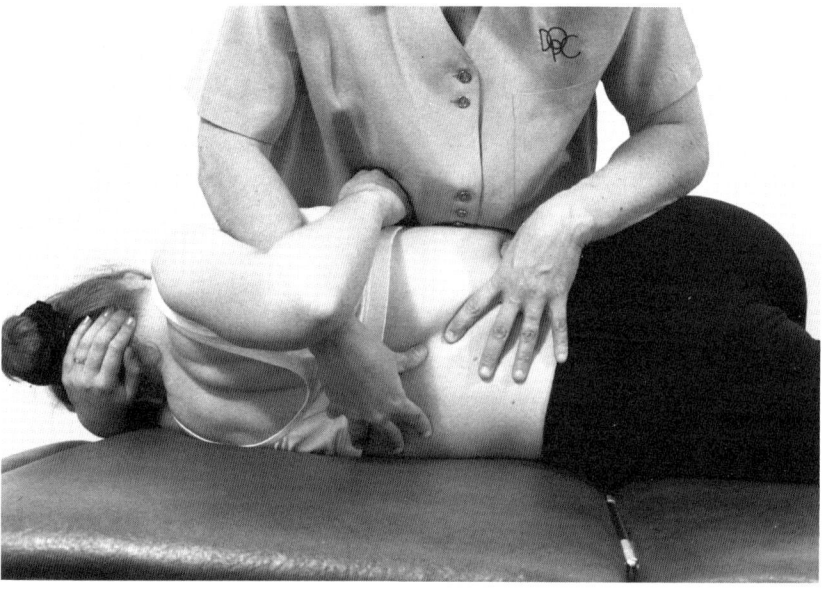

NOTES:

_____

_____

_____

_____

_____

_____

_____

Lumbar Region

LUMBAR REGION

ASSESSMENT

TREATMENT

POSITIONAL TESTS

Patient: Sitting, feet supported, or standing, feet directly under the hips, with even distribution of body weight through both lower limbs.

Therapist: Standing behind the patient.

Palpate: With the thumbs, palpate the articular pillars of the L3 vertebra.

Test: a) Flex the joint complex and assess the position of L3 relative to L4 by noting which articular pillar is the most dorsal. A dorsal left articular pillar of L3 relative to L4 is indicative of a left rotated position of the L3-4 joint complex in flexion.

b) Extend the joint complex and assess the position of the L3 vertebra relative to L4 by noting which articular pillar is the most dorsal. A dorsal left articular pillar of L3 relative to L4 is indicative of a left rotated position of the L3-4 joint complex in extension.

Addendum: This test may be performed with the patient prone, but in sitting or standing one can better observe the effect of the weight of the upper body on the joint mechanics.

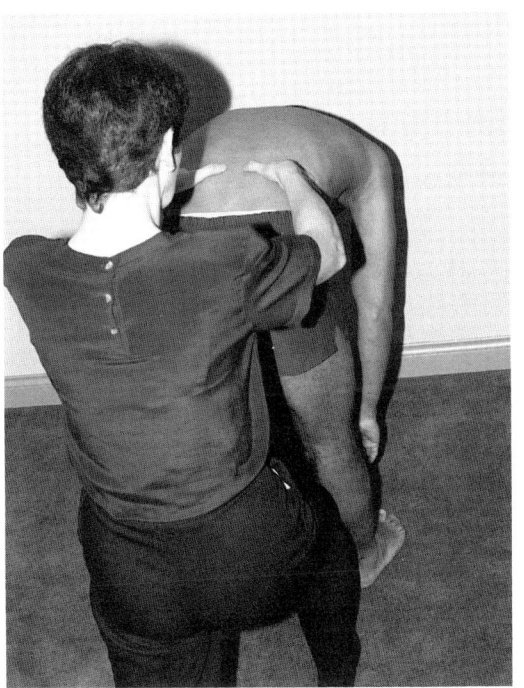

a) Flexion

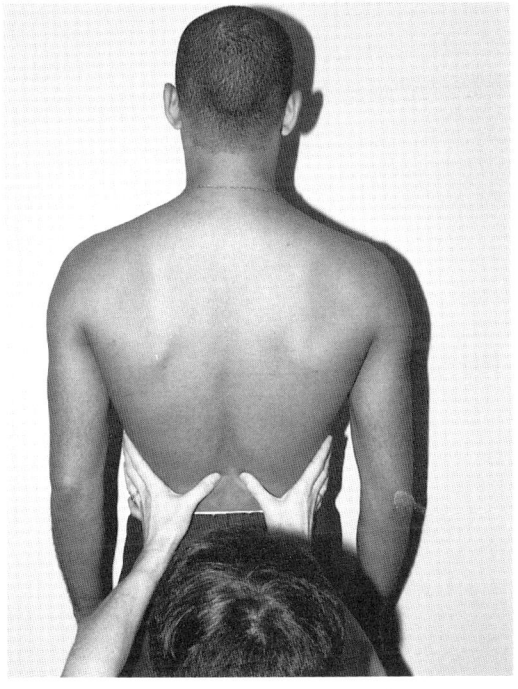

b) Extension

NOTES:

_____

_____

_____

ACTIVE MOBILITY TESTS OF OSTEOKINEMATIC FUNCTION

Forward bending

Patient:	Sitting, feet supported, or standing, feet directly under the hips, with even distribution of body weight through both lower limbs.
Therapist:	Standing behind the patient.
Palpate:	With the index finger and thumb of both hands, palpate the articular pillars of two adjacent vertebrae.
Test:	Instruct the patient to forward bend the lumbar spine and note the quantity, quality and symmetry of motion during flexion. Both index fingers should travel superoanteriorly an equal distance. When interpreting the mobility findings, the position of the joint at the beginning of the test should be correlated with the subsequent mobility noted since alterations in joint mobility may merely be a reflection of an altered starting position.

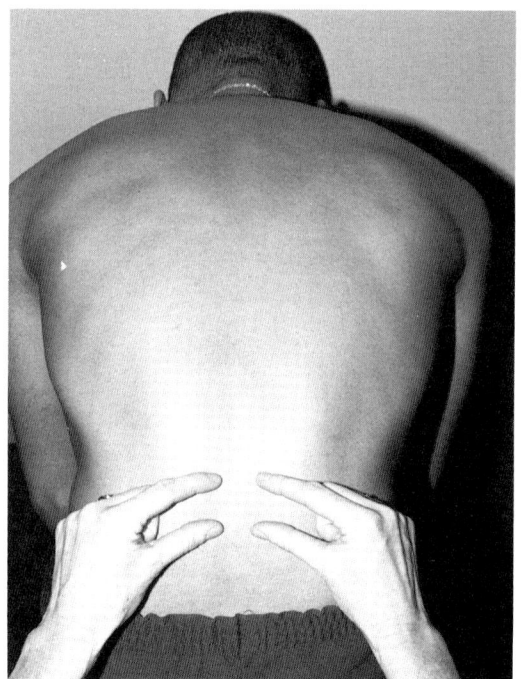

NOTES:

_____

_____

_____

_____

ACTIVE MOBILITY TESTS OF OSTEOKINEMATIC FUNCTION

Backward bending

Patient:	Sitting, feet supported, or standing, feet directly under the hips, with even distribution of body weight through both lower limbs.
Therapist:	Standing behind the patient.
Palpate:	With the index finger and thumb of both hands, palpate the articular pillars of two adjacent vertebrae.
Test:	Instruct the patient to backward bend the lumbar spine and note the quantity, quality and symmetry of motion during extension. Both index fingers should travel inferoposteriorly an equal distance. When interpreting the mobility findings, the position of the joint at the beginning of the test should be correlated with the subsequent mobility noted since alterations in joint mobility may merely be a reflection of an altered starting position.
Addendum:	This test may also be performed with the patient in prone, but in sitting or standing one can better observe the effect of the weight of the upper body on the joint mechanics.

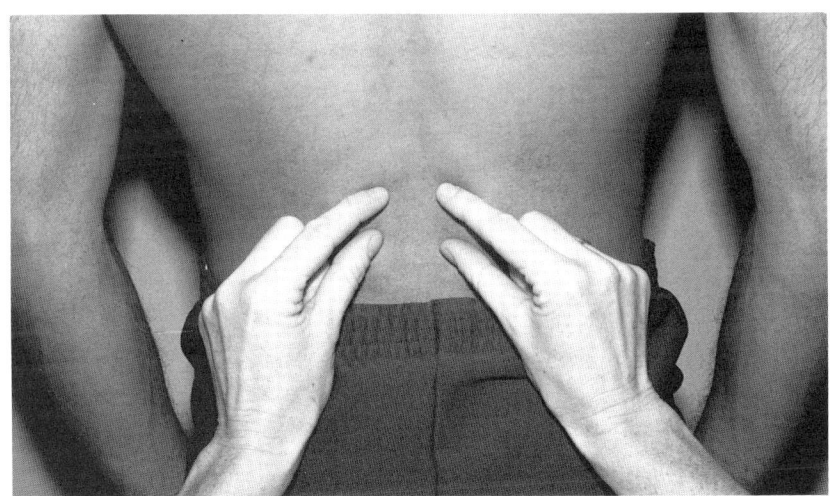

NOTES:
_____
_____
_____
_____
_____

ACTIVE MOBILITY TESTS OF OSTEOKINEMATIC FUNCTION

Lateral bending

Patient: Sitting, feet supported, or standing, feet directly under hips, with even distribution of body weight through both lower limbs.

Therapist: Standing behind the patient.

Palpate: With the index finger and thumb of both hands, palpate the articular pillars of two adjacent vertebrae.

Test: Instruct the patient to laterally bend the trunk and note the quantity, quality and direction of ease of motion. When interpreting the mobility findings, the position of the joint at the beginning of the test should be correlated with the subsequent mobility noted since alterations in joint mobility may merely be a reflection of an altered starting position.

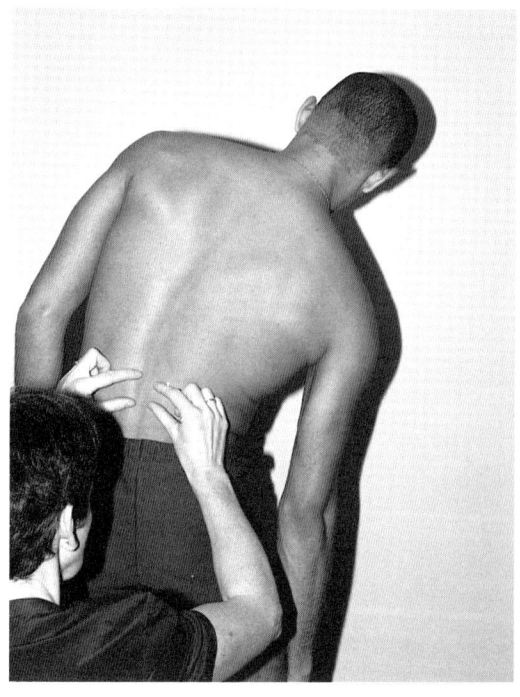

NOTES:

_____

_____

_____

_____

_____

ACTIVE MOBILITY TESTS OF OSTEOKINEMATIC FUNCTION

Rotation

Patient: Sitting, feet supported, or standing, feet directly under the hips, with even distribution of body weight through both lower limbs.

Therapist: Standing behind the patient.

Palpate: With the index finger and thumb of both hands, palpate the articular pillars of two adjacent vertebrae.

Test: Instruct the patient to rotate the lumbar spine and note the quantity, quality and direction of ease of motion. Also note whether lateral bending is ipsilateral or contralateral. When interpreting the mobility findings, the position of the joint at the beginning of the test should be correlated with the subsequent mobility noted since alterations in joint mobility may merely be a reflection of an altered starting position.

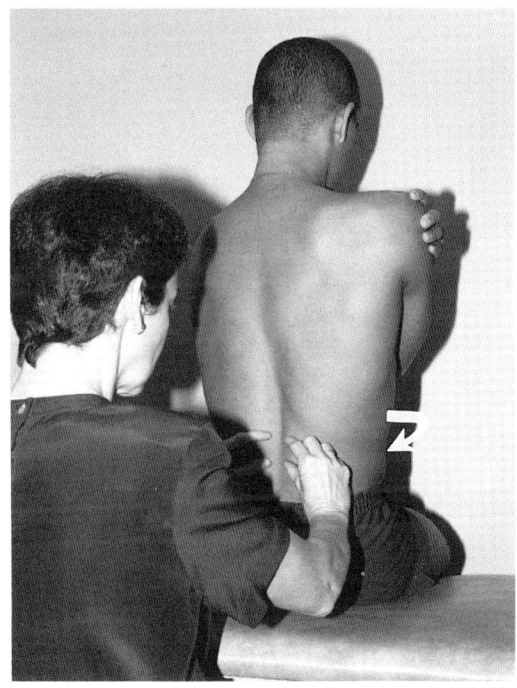

NOTES:

_____

_____

_____

_____

_____

_____

PASSIVE MOBILITY TESTS OF OSTEOKINEMATIC FUNCTION

Forward bending – sitting

Patient: Sitting, feet supported, arms crossed such that one arm is placed on the patient's abdomen, while the other hand rests on the opposite shoulder.

Therapist: Standing at the patient's side.

Palpate: With the index and long finger of the dorsal hand, palpate the articular pillars of the caudal vertebra of the segment being assessed. With the ventral hand, palpate the lumbar region at the level of the cranial vertebra of the segment being assessed, the ventral forearm resting on the patient's arm and abdomen.

Test: Fix L4 and passively flex (arrow) the L3-4 joint complex about the appropriate axis. Note the quantity, quality, direction of ease and the end feel of motion.

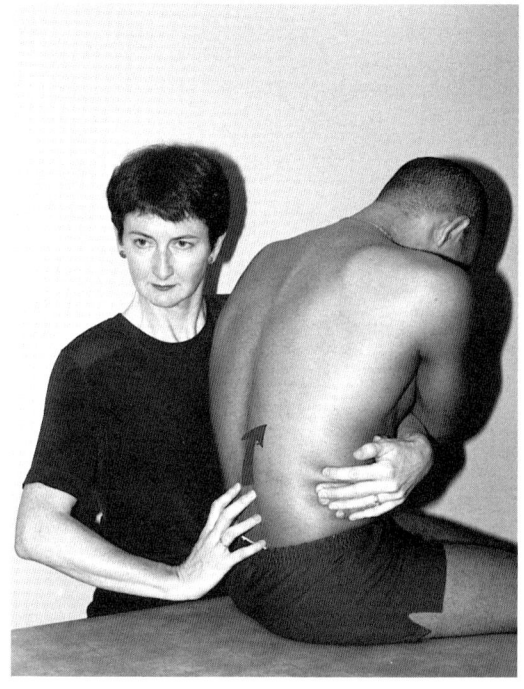

NOTES:

_____

_____

_____

_____

_____

PASSIVE MOBILITY TESTS OF OSTEOKINEMATIC FUNCTION

Forward bending – side lying

Patient: Side lying, lumbar spine supported in a neutral position, head resting on a pillow.

Therapist: Standing facing the patient.

Palpate: With the index and long finger of the caudal hand, palpate the interlaminar spaces of the joint complex being assessed. The forearm supports the lower lumbar spine and pelvic girdle. The therapist's lower thorax supports the patient's abdomen and iliac crest. With the cranial hand, palpate the cranial vertebra of the joint complex being assessed.

Test: Passively flex the joint complex by pushing the cranial vertebra superoanteriorly (arrow), using the therapist's cranial hand and forearm, thus flexing the joint complex. Note the quantity, quality, direction of ease and the end feel of motion.

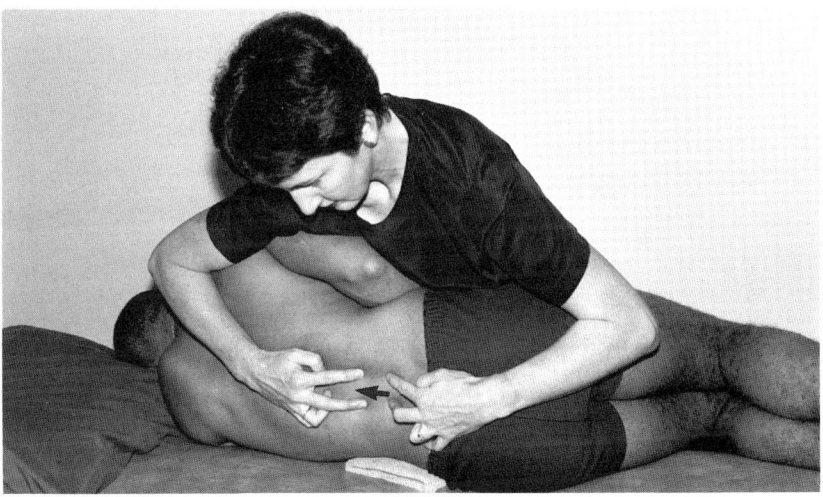

NOTES:

_____

_____

_____

_____

_____

_____

_____

PASSIVE MOBILITY TESTS OF OSTEOKINEMATIC FUNCTION

Backward bending – sitting

Patient:	Sitting, feet supported, arms crossed such that one arm is placed on the patient's abdomen, while the other hand rests on the opposite shoulder.
Therapist:	Standing at the patient's side.
Palpate:	With the index and long finger of the dorsal hand, palpate the articular pillars of the caudal vertebra of the segment being assessed. With the ventral hand, palpate the lumbar region at the level of the cranial vertebra of the segment being assessed, the ventral forearm resting on the patient's arm and abdomen.
Test:	Passively extend (arrow) the joint complex around the appropriate axis. Note the quantity, quality, direction of ease and the end feel of motion.

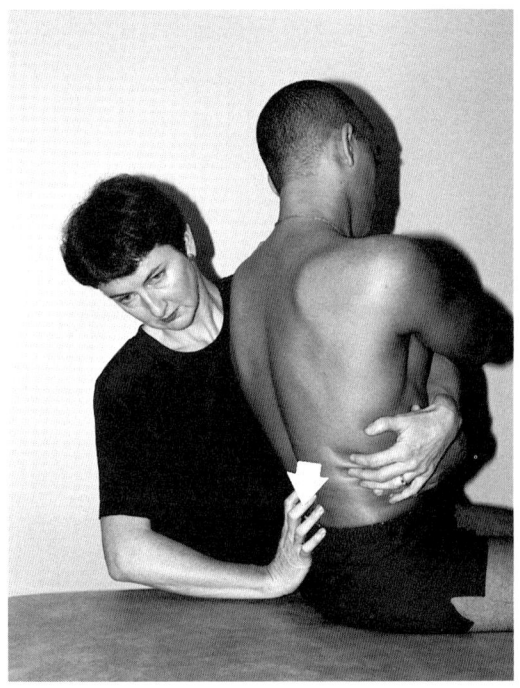

NOTES:

_____

_____

_____

_____

_____

PASSIVE MOBILITY TESTS OF OSTEOKINEMATIC FUNCTION

Backward bending – side lying

Patient:	Side lying, lumbar spine supported in a neutral position, head resting on a pillow.
Therapist:	Standing facing the patient.
Palpate:	With the index and long finger of the caudal hand, palpate the articular pillars of the caudal vertebra of the segment being assessed. The forearm supports the lower lumbar spine and the pelvic girdle. The therapist's lower thorax supports the patient's abdomen and anterior iliac crest. With the cranial hand, palpate the interlaminar space of the joint complex being assessed. The cranial forearm supports the patient's arm.
Test:	Passively extend the joint complex by pushing the caudal vertebra anteriorly (arrow), using the fingers of the caudal hand, thus extending the joint complex. The caudal forearm and therapist's lower thorax guides the anterior roll/translation of the caudal vertebra. Note the quantity, quality, direction of ease and the end feel of motion.

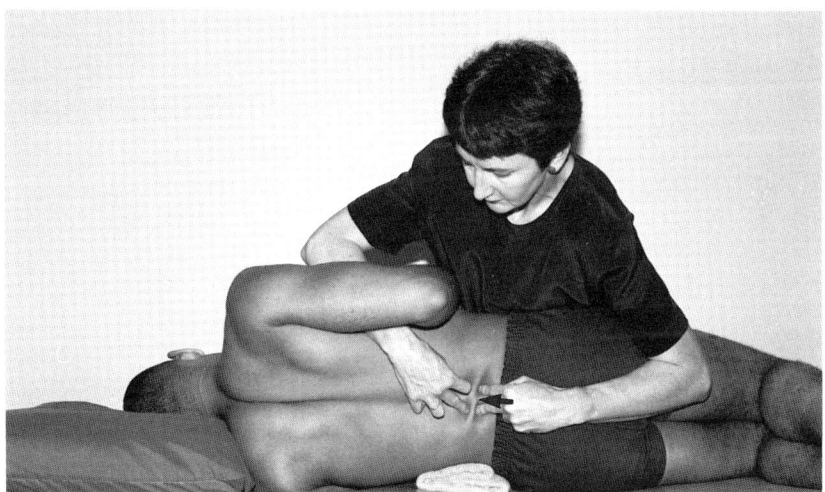

NOTES:

_____

_____

_____

_____

_____

PASSIVE MOBILITY TESTS OF OSTEOKINEMATIC FUNCTION

Lateral bending/rotation – sitting

Patient: Sitting, feet supported, arms crossed such that one arm is placed on the patient's abdomen, while the other hand rests on the opposite shoulder.

Therapist: Standing at the patient's side.

Palpate: With the index and long finger of the dorsal hand, palpate the interlaminar space of the segment. With the ventral hand, palpate the lumbar region at the level of the cranial vertebra, the ventral forearm resting on the patient's arm and abdomen.

Test: Passively laterally bend/rotate (arrow) the segment around the appropriate axis, observing whether ipsilateral or contralateral coupled motion occurs. Note the quantity, quality, direction of ease and the end feel of motion. This test may be performed in varying degrees of flexion and extension. Compare the findings in each position.

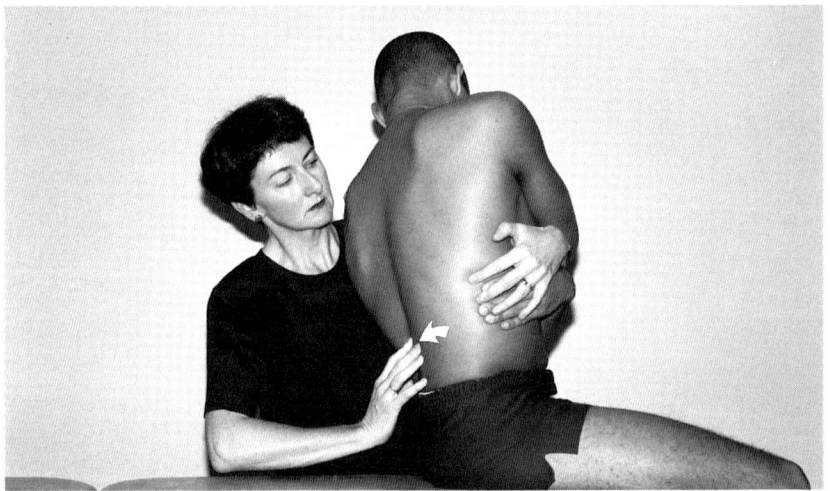

NOTES:

_____

_____

_____

_____

_____

_____

PASSIVE MOBILITY TESTS OF OSTEOKINEMATIC FUNCTION

Lateral bending/rotation – side lying

Patient: Side lying, lumbar spine supported in a neutral position, head resting on a pillow.

Therapist: Standing facing the patient.

Palpate: With the index and long finger of the caudal hand, palpate the interlaminar spaces of the segment being assessed. The forearm supports the lower lumbar spine and pelvic girdle. With the thumb of the cranial hand, palpate the lateral aspect (top) of the spinous process of the cranial vertebra. The cranial forearm supports the patient's arm.

Test: With the cranial forearm and thumb passively laterally bend/rotate (arrow) the segment around the appropriate axis, observing the presence of either ipsilateral or contralateral coupled motion. Note the quantity, quality, direction of ease and the end feel of motion. This test may be performed in varying degrees of flexion and extension. Compare the findings in each position.

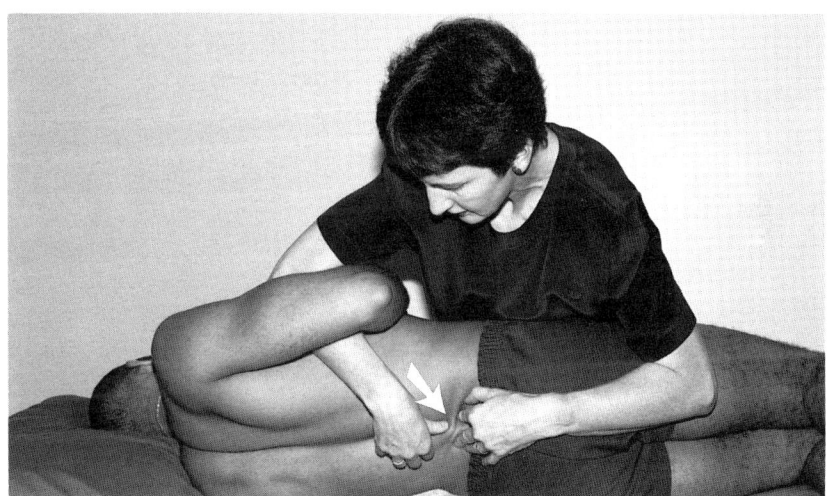

NOTES:

_____

_____

_____

_____

_____

_____

PASSIVE MOBILITY TESTS OF ARTHROKINEMATIC FUNCTION

Superoanterior glide – right zygapophysial joint L3-4

Patient: Prone, lumbar spine (especially the L3-4 segment) flexed to the motion barrier, using a pillow under the abdomen.

Therapist: Standing at the patient's side.

Palpate: With the index and long finger of one hand, palpate the articular pillars of L4. With the thumb of the other hand, palpate the right articular pillar of L3.

Test: Fix L4 and apply a force (arrow), varying the mediolateral inclination, to the right articular pillar of L3 to produce a superoanterior glide of the right zygapophysial joint at L3-4. Note the quantity, direction of ease and the end feel of motion.

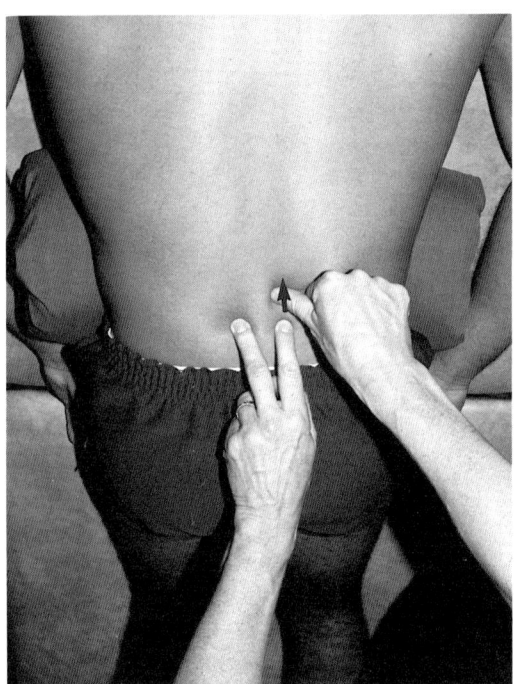

NOTES:

_____

_____

_____

_____

_____

_____

PASSIVE MOBILITY TESTS OF ARTHROKINEMATIC FUNCTION

Inferoposterior glide – left zygapophysial joint L3-4

Patient: Prone, lumbar spine (especially the L3-4 segment) extended to the motion barrier.

Therapist: Standing at the patient's side.

Palpate: With the index and long finger of the caudal hand, palpate the articular pillars of L4. With the thumb of the cranial hand, palpate the left articular pillar of L3.

Test: Fix L4 by applying a posteroanterior force to the articular pillars. Apply a force (arrow), varying the mediolateral inclination, to the left articular pillar of L3 to produce an inferoposterior glide of the right zygapophysial joint at L3-4. Note the quantity, quality, direction of ease and the end feel of motion.

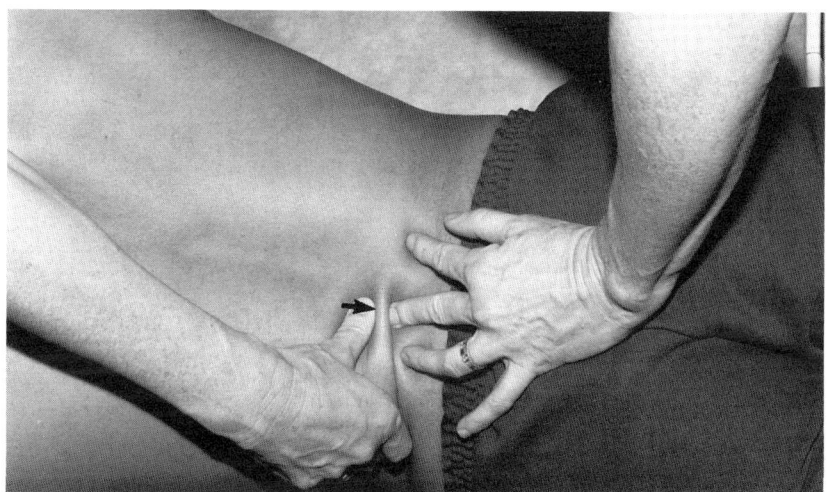

NOTES:

_____

_____

_____

_____

_____

_____

_____

_____

_____

PASSIVE MOBILITY TESTS OF ARTHROKINEMATIC FUNCTION

Right lateral translation L3-4

Patient:	Sitting, feet supported, arms crossed such that one arm is placed on the patient's abdomen, while the other hand rests on the opposite shoulder.
Therapist:	Standing facing the patient's right side.
Palpate:	With a lumbrical grip of the thumb and index finger of the dorsal hand, fix the L4 vertebra. With the ventral hand, palpate the lumbar region at the L3 level, the forearm rests over the patient's arm and abdomen.
Test:	Fix L4 and apply a right lateral translation force (arrow) to the L3-4 joint complex. Note the quantity, quality, direction of ease and the end feel of motion.

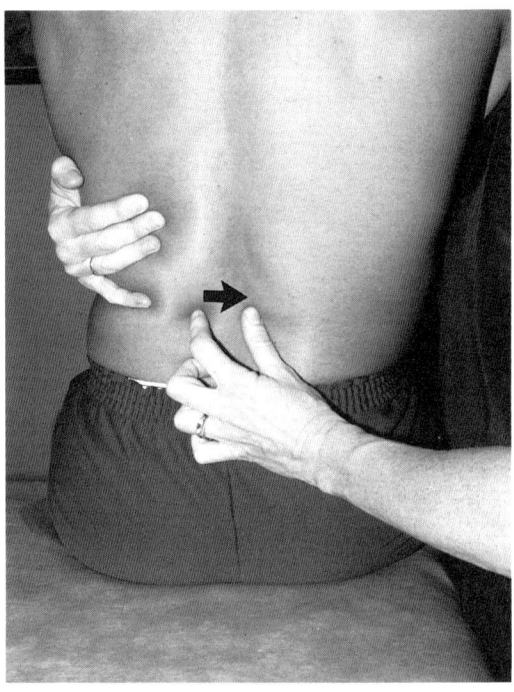

NOTES:

_____

_____

_____

_____

_____

_____

PASSIVE STABILITY TESTS OF ARTHROKINETIC FUNCTION

Vertical (compression)

Patient:	Supine, hips and knees flexed.
Therapist:	Standing at the patient's side.
Palpate:	With the cranial arm, cradle the patients's knees in order to control the degree of hip and knee flexion. With the caudal forearm, palpate the posterior aspect of the patient's thighs proximally.
Test:	a) With the lumbar spine in a neutral position, apply a compressive force cranially (arrow) with the caudal forearm. The direction of the force should be parallel to the floor. Note the reproduction of any symptoms.
	b) Repeat the test with the lumbar spine fully flexed (arrow). Note the reproduction of any symptoms.
	c) Repeat the test with the lumbar spine fully extended (arrow). (A roll may be used under the lumbar spine in order to maintain full extension.) Note the reproduction of any symptoms.

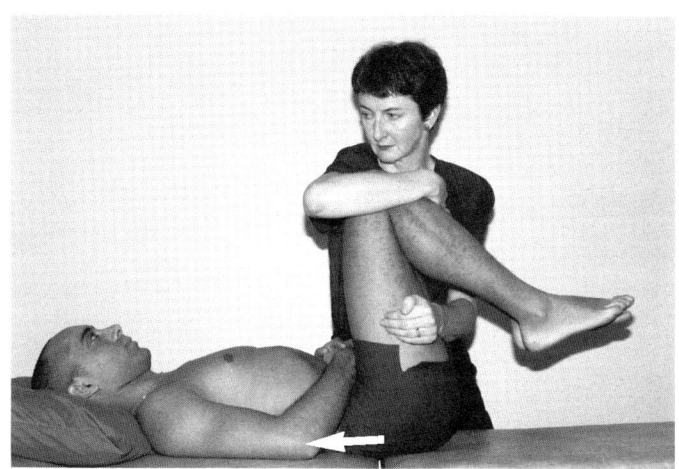

a) Neutral Compression

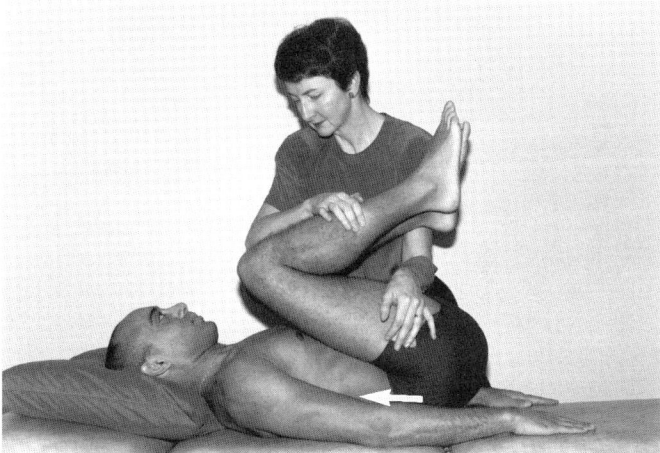

b) Compression in Flexion

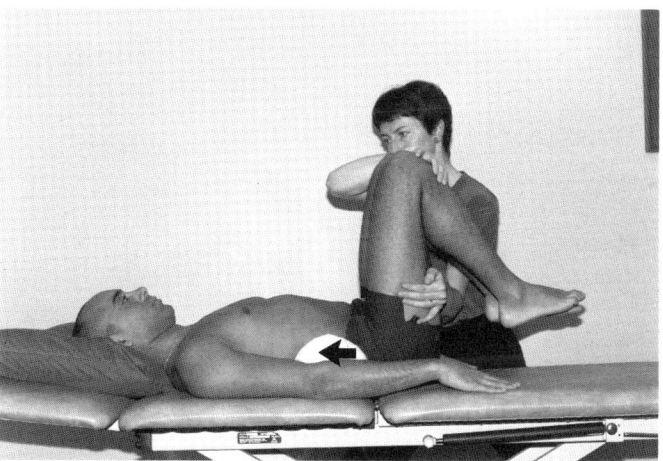

c) Compression in Extension

PASSIVE STABILITY TESTS OF ARTHROKINETIC FUNCTION

Vertical (traction)

Patient:	Supine, hips and knees flexed, feet placed close to the end of the table.
Therapist:	Standing at the end of the table facing the patient.
Palpate:	With the fingers interlaced, place the hands on the posterior aspect of the patient's proximal calves. A towel, wrapped around the patient's calves, may also be used.
Test:	Traction is applied (arrow) using a force in a caudal direction through the patient's calves. The angle of pull may be altered in accordance with the level being tested and the patient's response. Note the reproduction of any symptoms.

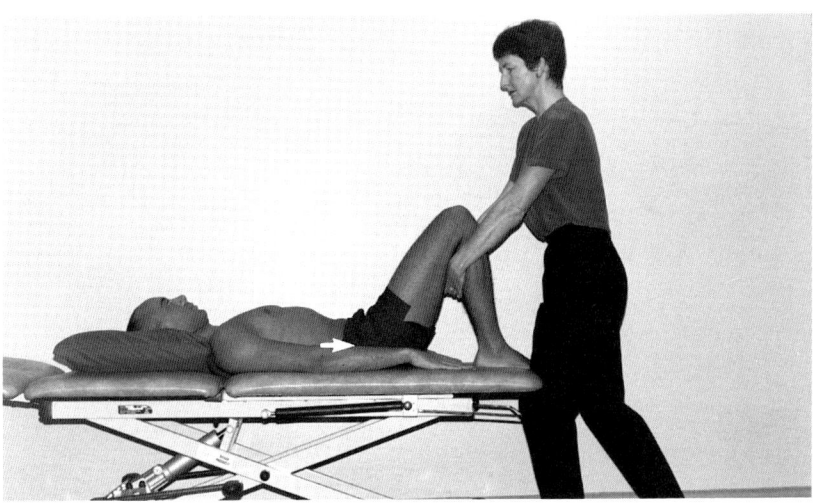

NOTES:

_____

_____

_____

_____

_____

_____

_____

_____

_____

PASSIVE STABILITY TESTS OF ARTHROKINETIC FUNCTION

Anterior translation L3-4

Patient:	Prone.
Therapist:	Standing at the patient's side.
Palpate:	With the index and long finger of the caudal hand, palpate the articular pillars of the L4 vertebra. With the pisiform and ulnar border of the cranial hand, palpate the spinous process of the L3 vertebra.
Test:	Fix L4 and apply a posteroanterior force to the L3 vertebra in a **PURE** horizontal plane (arrow). Sustain the force until the end feel is perceived. Note the quantity and end feel of motion as well as the reproduction of any symptoms.
Addendum:	The findings from this test should be correlated with those of the posterior translation test to determine the segmental level of instability.

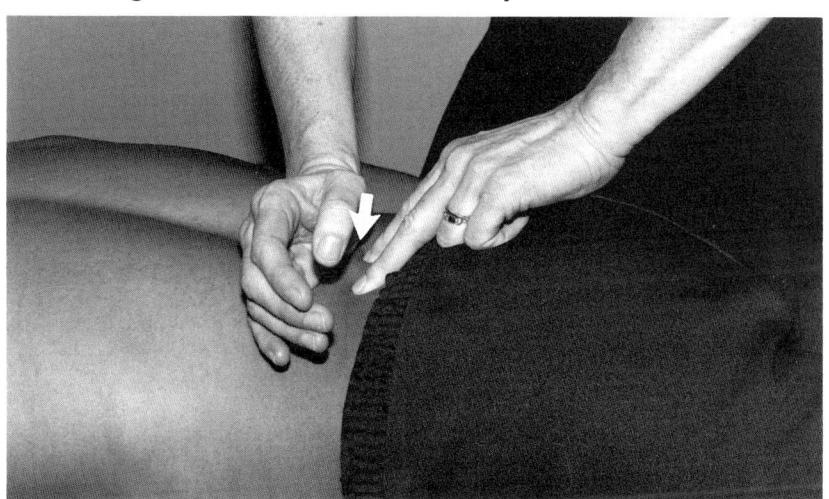

NOTES:

_____

_____

_____

_____

_____

_____

_____

_____

_____

PASSIVE STABILITY TESTS OF ARTHROKINETIC FUNCTION

Posterior translation L3-4 – sitting

Patient:	Sitting, arms crossed such that one arm is placed on the patient's abdomen, while the other hand rests on the opposite shoulder.
Therapist:	Standing at the patient's side.
Palpate:	With the dorsal hand, palpate the articular pillars of the L4 vertebra. With the ventral hand, palpate the lumbar region at the level of L3, the forearm rests over the patient's arm and abdomen.
Test:	Fix L4 and apply an anteroposterior force (arrow) to the L3 vertebra through the ventral forearm in a **PURE** horizontal plane. Sustain the force until the end feel is perceived. Note the quantity and end feel of motion as well as the reproduction of any symptoms.
Addendum:	The findings from this test should be correlated with those of the anterior translation test to determine the segmental level of instability.

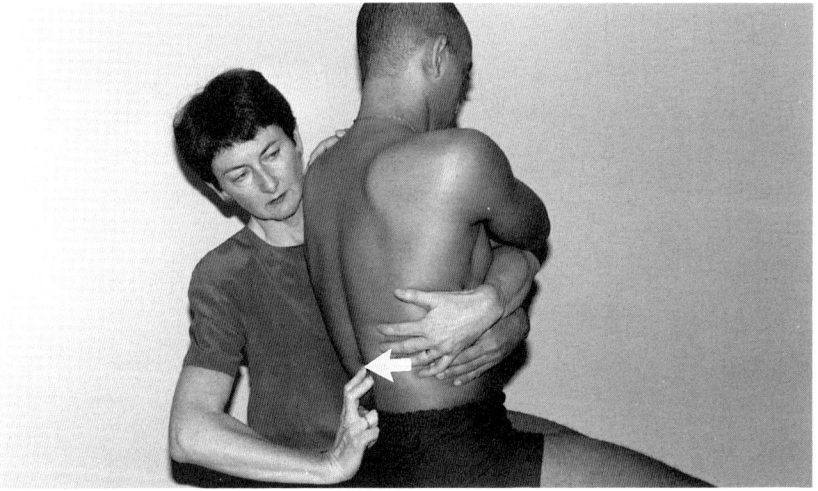

NOTES:

_____

_____

_____

_____

_____

_____

_____

PASSIVE STABILITY TESTS OF ARTHROKINETIC FUNCTION

Posterior translation L3-4 – prone

Patient:	Prone.
Therapist:	Standing at the patient's side.
Palpate:	With the index and long finger of the cranial hand, palpate the interlaminar spaces of L3-4. With the pisiform and ulnar border of the caudal hand, palpate the spinous process of the L4 vertebra.
Test:	Apply a posteroanterior force (arrow) to the L4 vertebra in a **PURE** horizontal plane, thus causing posterior translation of L3 on L4. Sustain the force until the end feel is perceived. Note the quantity and end feel of motion as well as the reproduction of any symptoms.
Addendum:	The findings from this test should be correlated with those of the anterior translation test to determine the segmental level of instability.

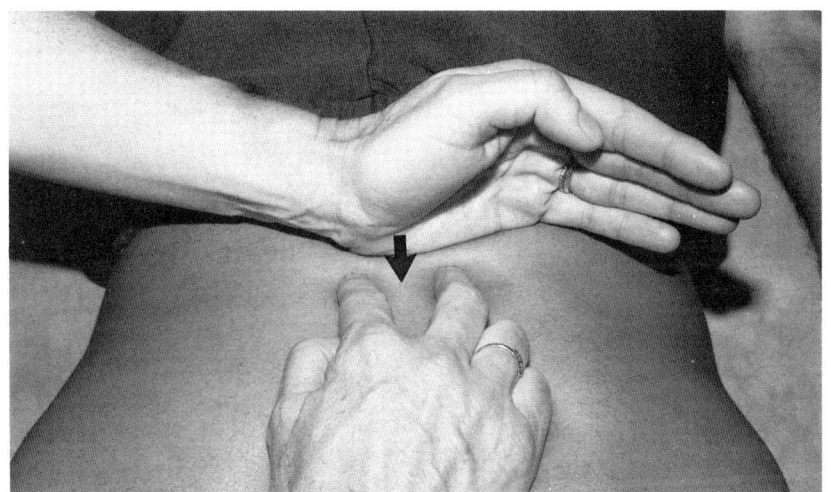

NOTES:

_____

_____

_____

_____

_____

_____

_____

_____

PASSIVE STABILITY TESTS OF ARTHROKINETIC FUNCTION

General torsion

Patient:	Prone.
Therapist:	Standing at the patient's side.
Palpate:	With the cranial hand, palpate the thoracolumbar junction. With the caudal hand, grasp the anterior aspect of the contralateral innominate bone.
Test:	Fix the thoracolumbar junction and apply a general torsion force (arrow) to the lumbar spine by lifting the contralateral innominate bone dorsally. Sustain the force until the end feel is perceived. Note the quantity and end feel of motion as well as the reproduction of any symptoms.

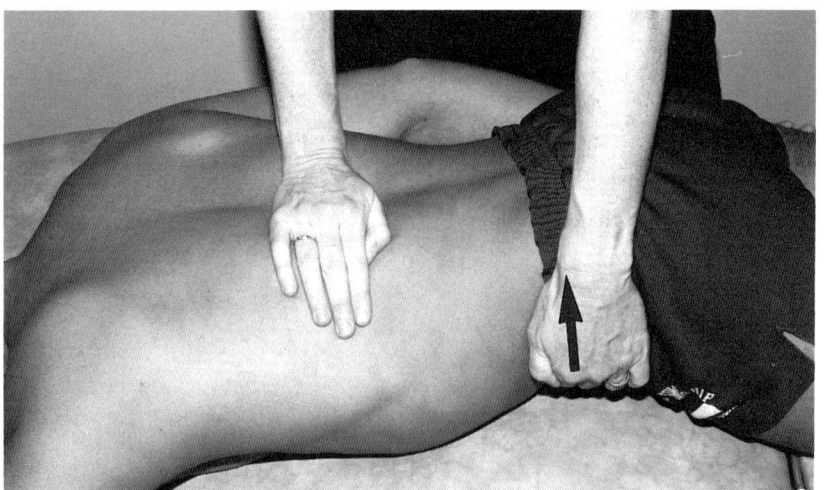

NOTES:

_____

_____

_____

_____

_____

_____

_____

_____

_____

_____

PASSIVE STABILITY TESTS OF ARTHROKINETIC FUNCTION

Left torsion L3-4

Patient: Right side lying, lumbar spine supported in a neutral position, head resting on a pillow.

Therapist: Standing facing the patient.

Palpate: With the thumb of the cranial hand, palpate the lateral aspect (top) of the spinous process of L3. The cranial forearm supports the patient's arm. With the index and long finger of the caudal hand, palpate the spinous process of L4 bilaterally. The therapist's forearm rests against the patient's pelvic girdle.

Test: Fix L4 and passively left rotate L3 (arrow) around a vertical axis using the cranial thumb. Sustain the force until the end feel is perceived. Note the quantity and end feel of motion as well as the reproduction of any symptoms. Compare this test with rotation in the opposite direction and for each segment.

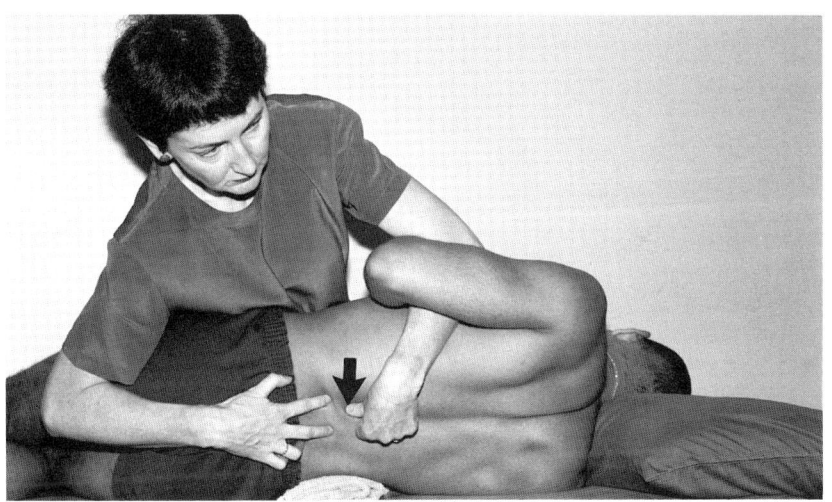

NOTES:

_____

_____

_____

_____

_____

_____

_____

PASSIVE STABILITY TESTS OF ARTHROKINETIC FUNCTION

Left lateral translation L3-4

Patient:	Left side lying.
Therapist:	Standing behind the patient.
Palpate:	With the radial border of the index finger of the caudal hand, palpate the lumbar region at the level of the left transverse process of L4. The ulnar border of this hand rests on the table, supporting the lumbar spine. With the pisiform and ulnar border of the cranial hand, palpate the lateral aspect of the right transverse process of L3.
Test:	Fix the L4 vertebra and apply a left lateral translation force (arrow) to the L3 vertebra with the cranial hand. Sustain the force until the end feel is perceived. Note the quantity and end feel of motion as well as the reproduction of any symptoms.

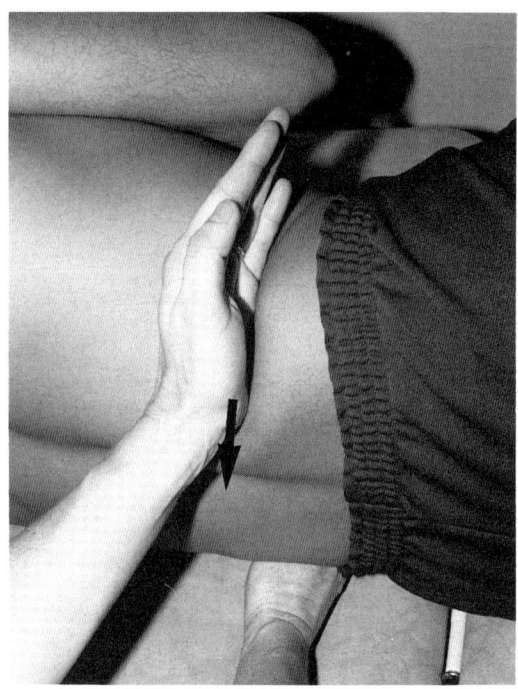

NOTES:

_____

_____

_____

_____

_____

PASSIVE STABILITY TESTS OF ARTHROKINETIC FUNCTION

Coronal plane stability – left iliolumbar ligament/lumbosacral junction

Patient:	Prone.
Therapist:	Standing at the patient's right side.
Palpate:	With the index and long finger of the cranial hand, palpate the articular pillars of the L5 vertebra. With the caudal hand, palpate the left aspect of the pelvic girdle or the lateral aspect of the left leg distal to the hip.
Test:	Fix the L5 vertebra and apply a lateral bending force, in the coronal plane (arrow), to the pelvic girdle until the motion barrier of right lateral bending at L5-S1 has been reached. Sustain the force until the end feel is perceived. Note the quantity and end feel of motion as well as the reproduction of any symptoms.

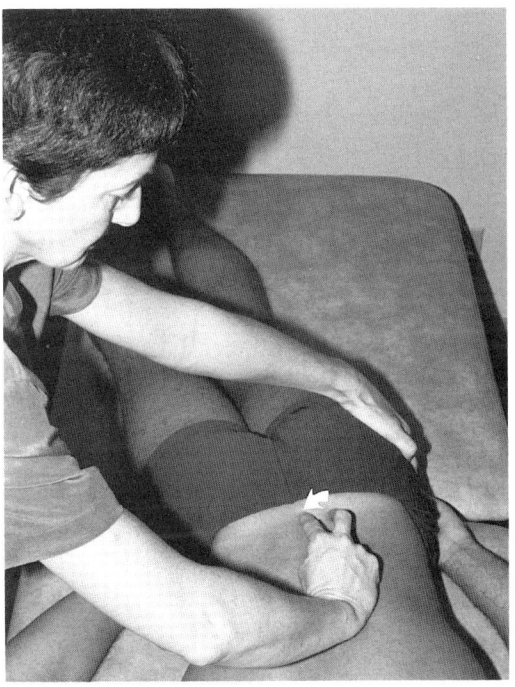

NOTES:

_____

_____

_____

_____

_____

PASSIVE STABILITY TESTS OF ARTHROKINETIC FUNCTION

Sagittal plane stability – right iliolumbar ligament/lumbosacral junction

Patient: Left side lying, left arm positioned posterior to the trunk and the right arm dangling towards the floor.

Therapist: Standing facing the patient.

Palpate: With the index and long finger of the caudal hand, palpate the sacral base. With the index finger of the cranial hand, palpate the lateral aspect (bottom) of the spinous process of L5.

Localization: Fix the sacrum and apply a left torsion force to the L5 vertebra. Ask the patient to assist by breathing out and allowing the right arm to dangle further towards the floor. This left rotation technique of the L5-S1 joint complex is repeated until the motion barrier for left rotation at the L5-S1 joint complex has been reached, thus increasing the distance between the right transverse process of L5 and the iliac crest.

Test: With the cranial hand, fix the trunk and the L5 vertebra in left rotation. With the caudal hand, apply an anteroposterior force (arrow) to the anterior aspect of the iliac crest, thus stressing the most sagitally oriented fibres of the right iliolumbar ligament. Sustain the force until the end feel is perceived. Note the quantity and end feel of motion as well as the reproduction of any symptoms.

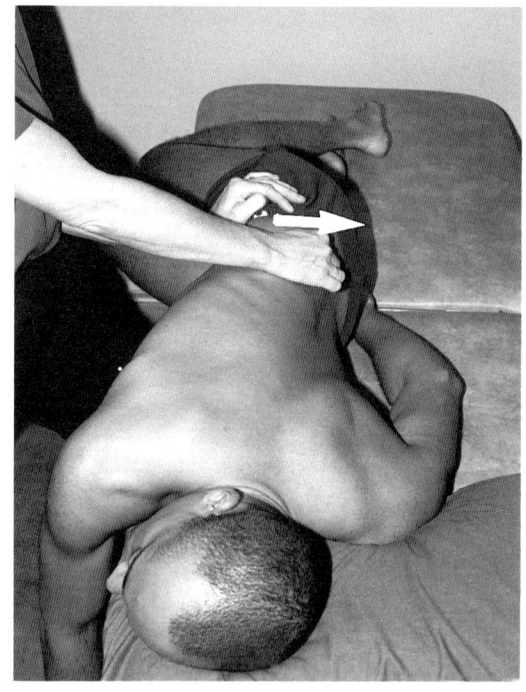

Assessment

MOBILIZATION TECHNIQUES

Restriction of flexion (superoanterior glide) L3-4

Patient: Side lying, lumbar spine supported in a neutral position, head resting on a pillow.

Therapist: Standing facing the patient.

Palpate: 1. With the index and long finger of the cranial hand, palpate the interlaminar spaces of the L3-4 joint complex. With the caudal hand, flex the hips, knees and the lower lumbar spine including L4-5, to the motion barrier, leaving the L3-4 joint complex in a neutral position. The patient's lower leg is then extended.

2. With the index and long finger of the caudal hand, palpate the interlaminar spaces of the L3-4 joint complex. With the cranial hand and forearm, lock the upper lumbar spine either congruently or incongruently with lateral bending and rotation in either neutral, flexion or extension by pulling through the patient's lower arm. The L3-4 joint complex remains in a neutral position.

Localization: Fix L4 and flex the L3-4 joint complex to the motion barrier using the cranial hand and forearm.

Mobilization: **Passive:** Apply a grade 1 to 4 force to produce a superoanterior glide (arrow) of the zygapophyseal joints at L3-4 using the cranial hand and forearm.

Active: From the motion barrier, instruct the patient to meet the therapist's resistance. The direction of resistance is that which facilitates further flexion at L3-4. The isometric contraction is held for up to 5 seconds and followed by a period of complete relaxation. The joint is then passively taken to the new motion barrier. This technique is repeated 3 times and followed by a re-evaluation of osteokinematic, arthrokinematic and arthrokinetic function.

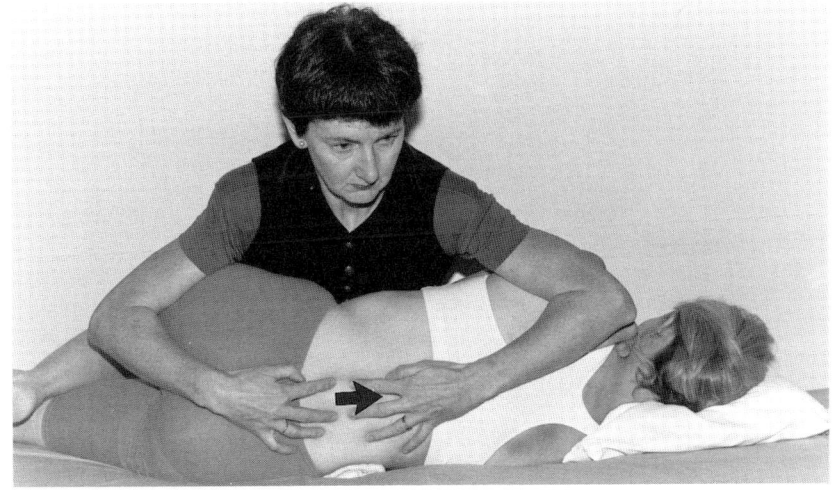

MOBILIZATION TECHNIQUES

Restriction of flexion/left lateral bending/rotation (superoanterior glide right zygapophysial joint) L3-4

Patient: Left side lying, lumbar spine supported in a neutral position, head resting on a pillow.

Therapist: Standing facing the patient.

Palpate: 1. With the index and long finger of the cranial hand, palpate the interlaminar spaces of the L3-4 joint complex. With the caudal hand, flex the hips, knees and the lower lumbar spine including L4-5 to the motion barrier, leaving the L3-4 joint complex in a neutral position. The patient's lower leg is then extended.

2. With the index and long finger of the caudal hand, palpate the interlaminar spaces of the L3-4 joint complex. With the cranial hand and forearm, lock the upper lumbar spine either congruently or incongruently using lateral bending and rotation in either neutral, flexion or extension by pulling through the patient's lower arm. The L3-4 joint complex remains in a neutral position.

Localization: Fix L4 with the caudal hand. Flex, left laterally bend and rotate the L3-4 joint complex to the motion barrier.

Mobilization: **Passive** – Apply a grade 1 to 5 force to produce a superoanterior glide (arrow) of the right zygapophysial joint at L3-4.

Active – From the motion barrier, instruct the patient to gently meet the therapist's resistance. The direction of resistance is that which facilitates further flexion, left lateral bending, rotation of the joint complex. The isometric contraction is held for up to 5 seconds and followed by a period of complete relaxation. The joint is then passively taken to the new motion barrier. This technique is repeated 3 times and followed by a re-evaluation of osteokinematic, arthrokinematic and arthrokinetic function.

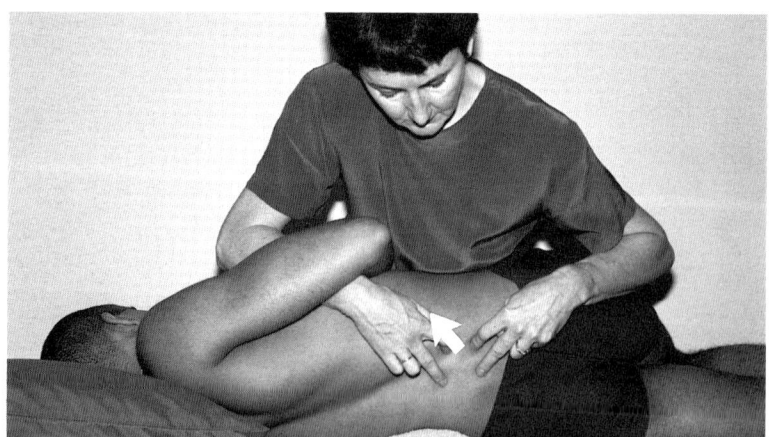

MOBILIZATION TECHNIQUES

Restriction of flexion/left lateral bending/rotation (superoanterior glide right zygapophysial joint) L5-S1

Patient:	Right side lying, lumbar spine supported in a neutral position, head resting on a pillow.
Therapist:	Standing facing the patient.
Palpate:	With the index and long finger of the cranial hand, palpate the interlaminar spaces of the L5-S1 joint complex. Flex the hips, knees and the sacroiliac joints to the motion barrier and then extend the patient's lower leg. The L5-S1 joint complex remains in a neutral position. The rest of the hand and forearm supports the pelvic girdle. The therapist's lower thorax supports the patient's iliac crest. The L4-5 joint complex is locked congruently or incongruently with lateral bending and rotation in neutral, flexion or extension by pulling through the patient's lower arm.
Localization:	Flex, left laterally bend, rotate the L5-S1 joint complex to the motion barrier, through the pelvic girdle, using the therapist's caudal arm and lower thorax.
Mobilization:	**Passive** – Apply a grade 1 to 5 force (arrow) to the pelvic girdle to produce a superoanterior glide of the right zygapophysial joint at L5-S1.
	Active – From the motion barrier, instruct the patient to gently meet the therapist's resistance. The direction of resistance is that which facilitates further flexion, left lateral bending, rotation. The isometric contraction is held for up to 5 seconds and followed by a period of complete relaxation. The joint is then passively taken to the new motion barrier. This technique is repeated 3 times and followed by a re-evaluation of osteokinematic, arthrokinematic and arthrokinetic function.

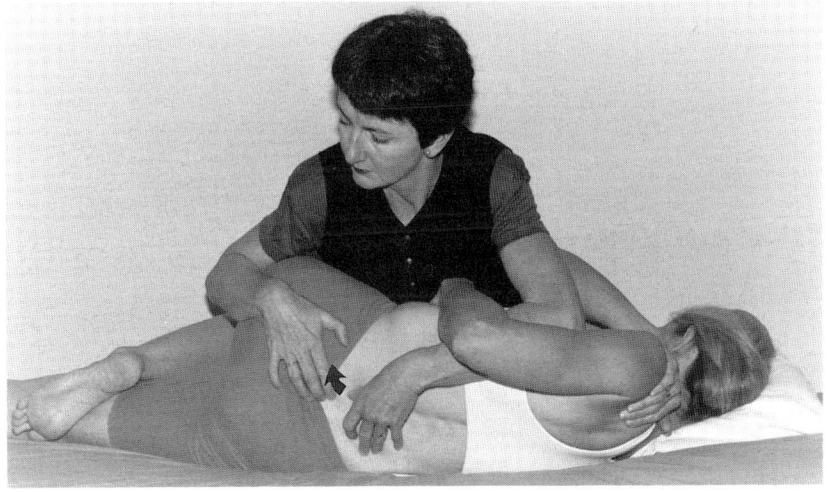

MOBILIZATION TECHNIQUES

Restriction of extension (posteroinferior glide) L3-4

Patient: Side lying, lumbar spine supported in a neutral position, head resting on a pillow.

Therapist: Standing facing the patient.

Palpate: 1. With the index and long finger of the cranial hand, palpate the interlaminar spaces of the L3-4 joint complex. With the caudal hand, extend the lower lumbar spine including L4-5, leaving the L3-4 joint complex in a neutral position. The patients upper hip and knee is flexed while the lower leg is extended.

2. With the index and long finger of the caudal hand, palpate the interlaminar spaces of the L3-4 joint complex. With the cranial hand and forearm, lock the upper lumbar spine either congruently or incongruently using lateral bending and rotation in either neutral, flexion or extension by pulling through the patient's lower arm. The L3-4 joint complex remains in a neutral position.

Localization: Fix L4 by applying a posteroanterior force to the articular pillars of the L4 vertebra using the index and long finger of the caudal hand.

Passive: Apply a grade 1 to 4 force to produce a posteroinferior glide (arrow) of the zygapophyseal joints at L3-4 using the cranial hand and forearm.

Mobilization: **Active** – From the motion barrier, instruct the patient to gently meet the therapist's resistance. The direction of resistance is that which facilitates extension. The isometric contraction is held for up to 5 seconds and followed by a period of complete relaxation. The joint is then passively taken to the new motion barrier. This technique is repeated 3 times and followed by a re-evaluation of osteokinematic, arthrokinematic and arthrokinetic function.

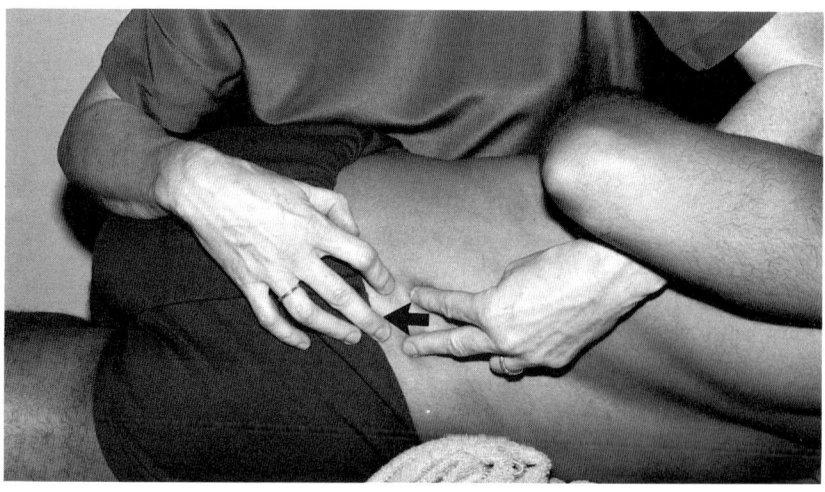

MOBILIZATION TECHNIQUES

Restriction of extension/right lateral bending/rotation (posteroinferior glide right zygapophysial joint) L3-4

Patient: Left side lying, lumbar spine supported in a neutral position, head resting on a pillow.

Therapist: Standing facing the patient.

Palpate: 1. With the index and long finger of the cranial hand, palpate the interlaminar spaces of the L3-4 joint complex. With the caudal hand, extend the lower lumbar spine, including L4-5, to the motion barrier, leaving the L3-4 joint complex in a neutral position. The patient's upper hip and knee is flexed while the hip and the knee of the lower leg is extended.

2. With the index and long finger of the caudal hand, palpate the interlaminar spaces of the L3-4 joint complex. With the cranial hand and forearm, lock the upper lumbar spine either congruently or incongruently using lateral bending and rotation in either neutral, flexion or extension by pulling through the patient's lower arm. The L3-4 joint complex remains in a neutral position.

Localization: Fix L4 by applying a posteroanterior force to the articular pillars using the index and long finger of the caudal hand. Extend, right laterally bend, rotate the L3-4 joint complex to the motion barrier using the cranial thumb applied to the inferior articular process of L3 and the cranial forearm applied to the lower lateral thorax.

Continued on Page 210

NOTES:

_____

_____

_____

_____

_____

_____

_____

_____

_____

_____

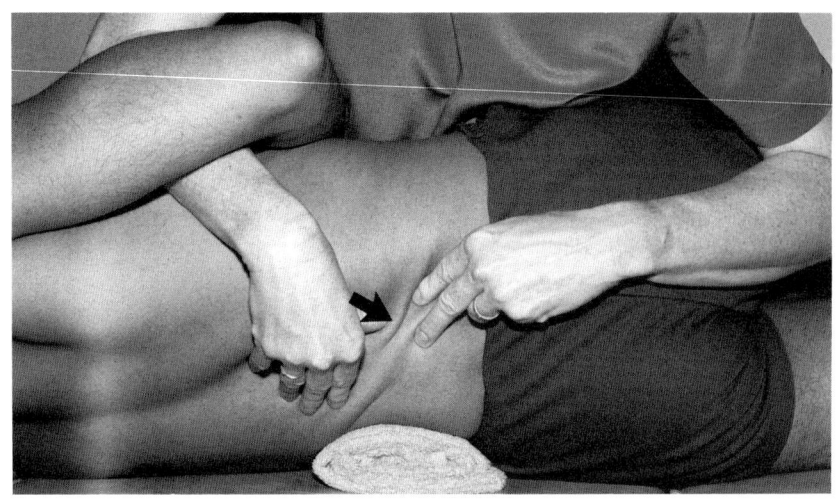

Mobilization: **Passive** – Apply a grade 1 to 5 force to produce a posteroinferior glide (arrow) of the right zygapophysial joint at L3-4.

Active – From the motion barrier, instruct the patient to gently meet the therapist's resistance. The direction of resistance is that which facilitates further extension, right lateral bending, rotation. The isometric contraction is held for up to 5 seconds and followed by a period of complete relaxation. The joint is then passively taken to the new motion barrier. This technique is repeated 3 times and followed by a re-evaluation of osteokinematic, arthrokinematic and arthrokinetic function.

NOTES:

_____

_____

_____

_____

_____

_____

_____

_____

_____

_____

_____

MOBILIZATION TECHNIQUES

General traction

Patient:	Supine, hips and knees flexed, feet placed close to the end of the table.
Therapist:	Standing at the end of the table facing the patient.
Palpate:	With the fingers interlaced, place the hands on the posterior aspect of the patient's proximal calves.
Localization:	Localization is achieved by varying the angle of pull through the patient's thighs, thus localizing the traction force to the upper, middle or lower lumbar region.
Mobilization:	A grade 1 to 4 longitudinal traction force (arrow) is applied to the lumbar spine by leaning backwards and pulling through the hands.

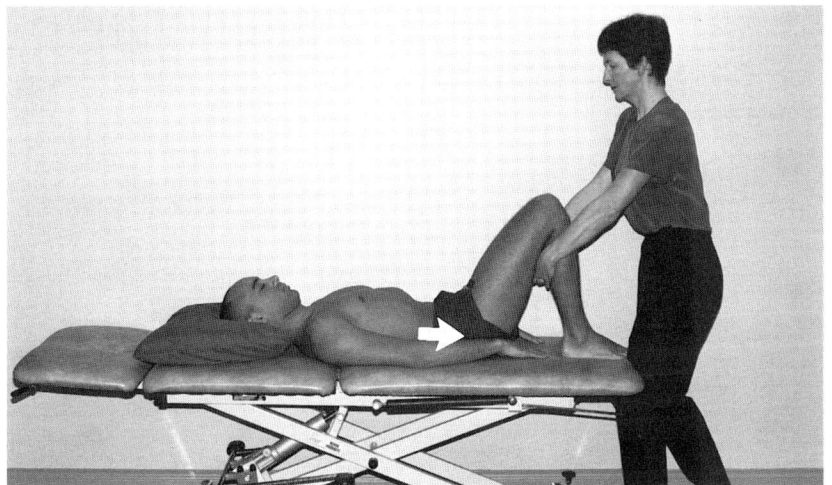

NOTES:

_____

_____

_____

_____

_____

_____

_____

_____

_____

_____

MOBILIZATION TECHNIQUES

Specific traction L3-4

Patient:	Side lying, lumbar spine supported in a neutral position, head resting on a pillow.
Therapist:	Standing facing the patient.
Palpate:	1. With the index and long finger of the caudal hand, palpate the interlaminar spaces of the L3-4 joint complex. The patient's upper hip and knee is flexed while the lower hip and knee is extended. Lock the upper lumbar spine either congruently or incongruently with lateral bending and rotation in either neutral, flexion or extension by pulling through the patient's lower arm. The L3-4 joint complex remains in a neutral position.
	2. With the index and long finger of the cranial hand, palpate the interlaminar spaces of the L3-4 joint complex. With the caudal hand flex the lower lumbar spine to the motion barrier. The L3-4 joint complex remains in neutral.
Localization:	Fix L3 by applying a posteroanterior force to the articular pillars of the L3 vertebra, using the index and long finger of the cranial hand. With the caudal hand, palpate the interlaminar space of the L3-4 joint complex. The rest of this hand and forearm rests on the patient's pelvic girdle. The therapist's lower lateral thorax is applied to the anterosuperior aspect of the patient's iliac crest.
Mobilization:	Apply a grade 1 to 4 longitudinal traction force (arrow) to the L3-4 joint complex through the patient's pelvic girdle using the caudal hand, forearm and the lower lateral thorax.

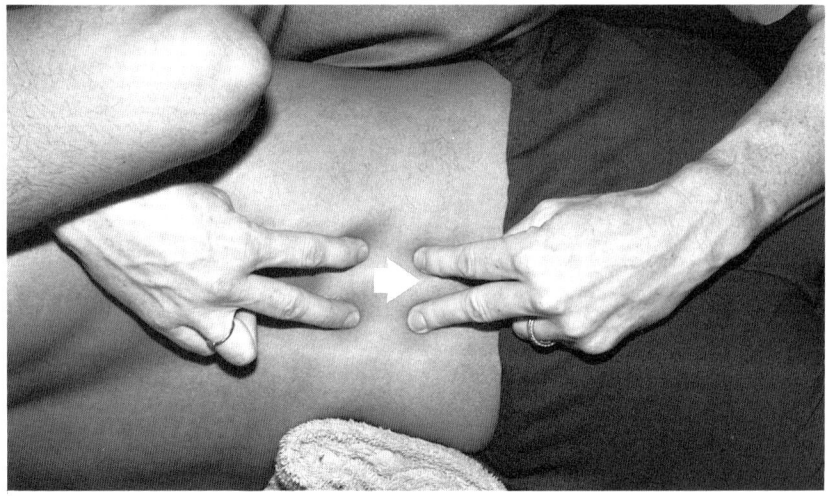

MOBILIZATION TECHNIQUES

Restriction of right lateral translation L5-S1

Patient: Standing, feet placed apart for stability.

Therapist: Standing at the patient's right side facing the patient.

Palpate: With the index and long finger of the dorsal hand, palpate the sacral base. The ventral forearm supports the abdomen while the ventral hand is placed on the lumbar region at the level of the L5 vertebra. The therapist's right side is placed against the patient's right iliac crest.

Localization: With the dorsal hand and the therapist's right side, fix the patient's pelvic girdle.

Mobilization: Apply a right lateral translation force (arrow) to the L5-S1 joint complex using the right hand and forearm.
Caution: avoid causing muscle spasm or peripheralization of symptoms.

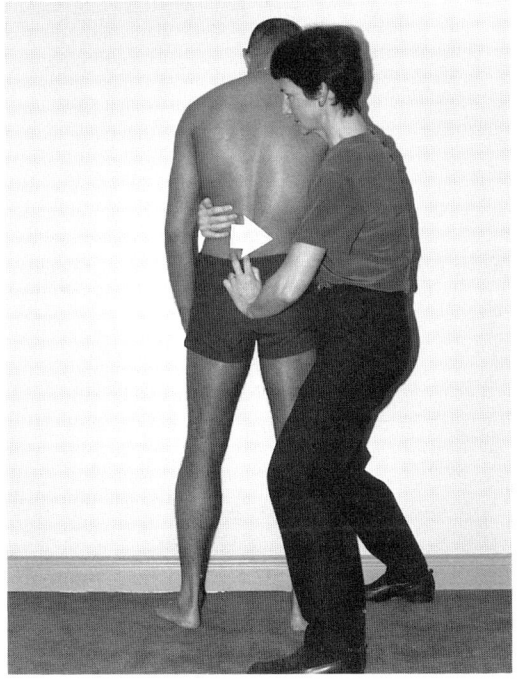

NOTES:

_____

_____

_____

_____

_____

MOBILIZATION TECHNIQUES

Restriction of longitudinal soft tissue mobility

Patient: Side lying, lumbar spine supported on a pillow.

Therapist: Standing facing the patient.

Palpate: With the forearms resting on the patient's lateral thorax and pelvic girdle and the fingers flexed in a lumbrical grip, palpate the soft tissue of the uppermost side.

Localization: The soft tissue slack is taken up as the therapist simultaneously adducts the shoulders and flexes the elbows while maintaining the hands in a loose lumbrical grip.

Mobilization: Apply a longitudinal mobilization force to the soft tissue (arrow), resulting in a longitudinal stretch of this tissue.

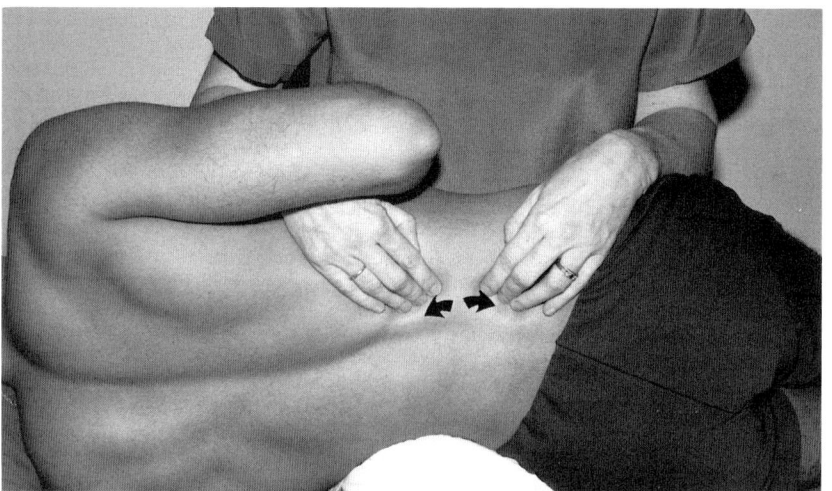

NOTES:

_____

_____

_____

_____

_____

_____

_____

_____

_____

_____

Pelvic Girdle

PELVIC GIRDLE

ASSESSMENT

TREATMENT

POSITIONAL TESTS — INNOMINATE

Iliac crest

Patient: Supine.
Therapist: Standing at the patient's side.
Palpate: With the radial border of the index fingers, palpate the lateral aspect of the iliac crests. Move the soft tissue overlying the iliac crest medially and so that the index fingers rest on the highest point of the iliac crest. Using peripheral vision, compare the craniocaudal relationship of the two sides.

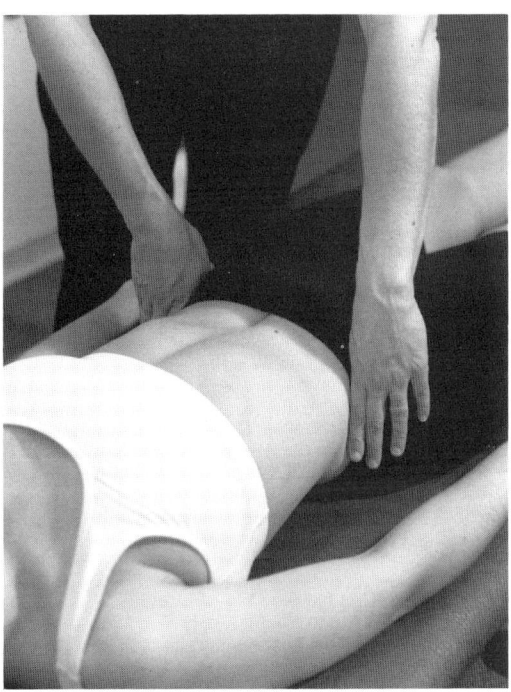

NOTES:

_____

_____

_____

_____

_____

_____

_____

_____

POSITIONAL TESTS — INNOMINATE

Anterior Superior Iliac Spine

Patient:	Supine.
Therapist:	Standing at the patient's side.
Palpate:	Initially, palpate the anterior superior iliac spine (ASIS) through the soft tissue with the heel of the hand.

Then using the thumbs,

1. Palpate the inferior aspect of the ASIS's. Using peripheral vision, compare the craniocaudal relationship of the two sides.

2. Palpate the medial aspect of the ASIS's. Using peripheral vision, compare the mediolateral relationship of the ASIS to the midline of the body.

3. Palpate the ventral aspect of the ASIS's. Compare the anteroposterior relationship of the two sides.

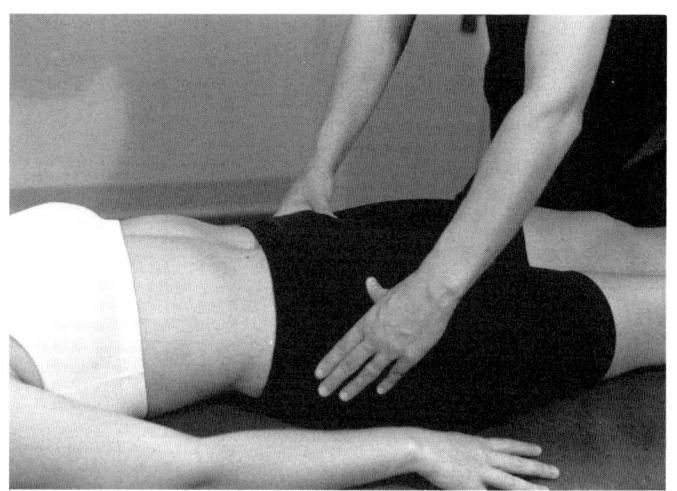 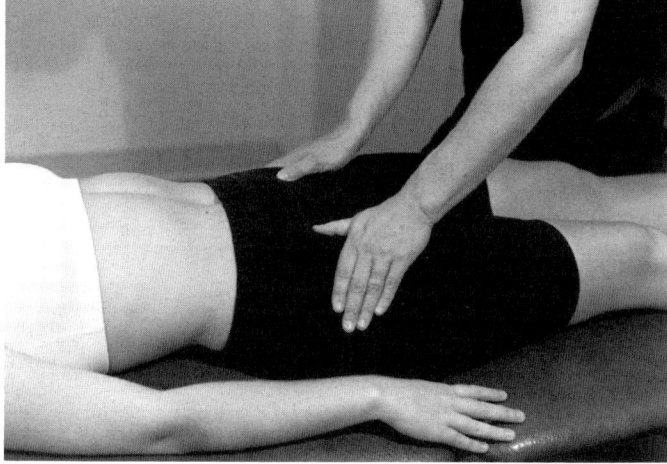

NOTES:

_____

_____

_____

_____

_____

_____

POSITIONAL TESTS — INNOMINATE

Pubic Tubercle

Patient: Supine.
Therapist: Standing at the patient's side.
Palpate: Initially, palpate the pubic symphysis through the soft tissue with the heel of the hand.

Then using the thumbs,

1. Palpate the superior aspect of the pubic tubercles which are approximately 1 cm apart and superior to the symphysis. Compare the craniocaudal relationship of the two sides.

2. Palpate the ventral aspect of the pubic tubercles. Compare the anteroposterior relationship of the two sides.

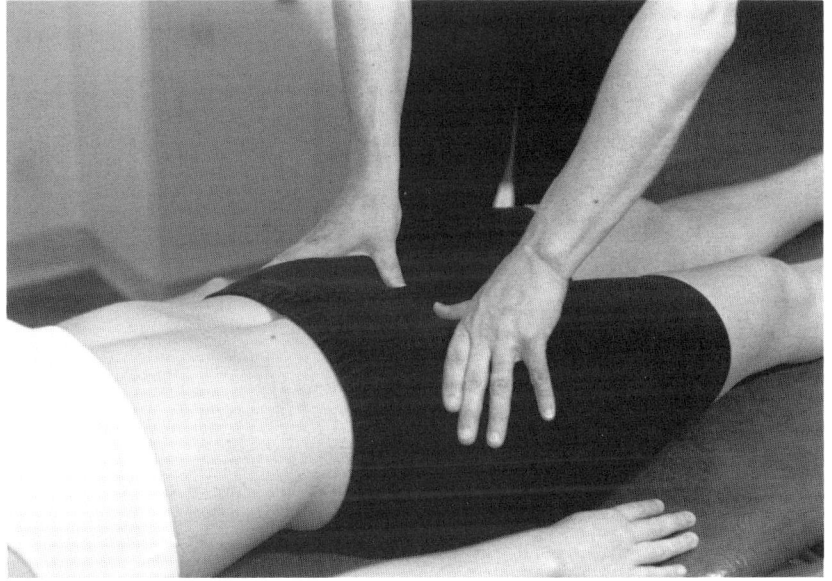

NOTES:

_____

_____

_____

_____

_____

_____

POSITIONAL TESTS — INNOMINATE

Posterior Superior Iliac Spine

Patient: Prone.
Therapist: Standing at the patient's side.
Palpate: Observe the 'dimple'. The PSIS lies approximately 1 cm inferior to the dimple.

Then using the thumbs,

1. Palpate the inferior aspect of the PSIS's. Using peripheral vision, compare the craniocaudal relationship of the two sides.

2. Palpate the dorsal aspect of the PSIS's. Compare the anteroposterior relationship of the two sides.

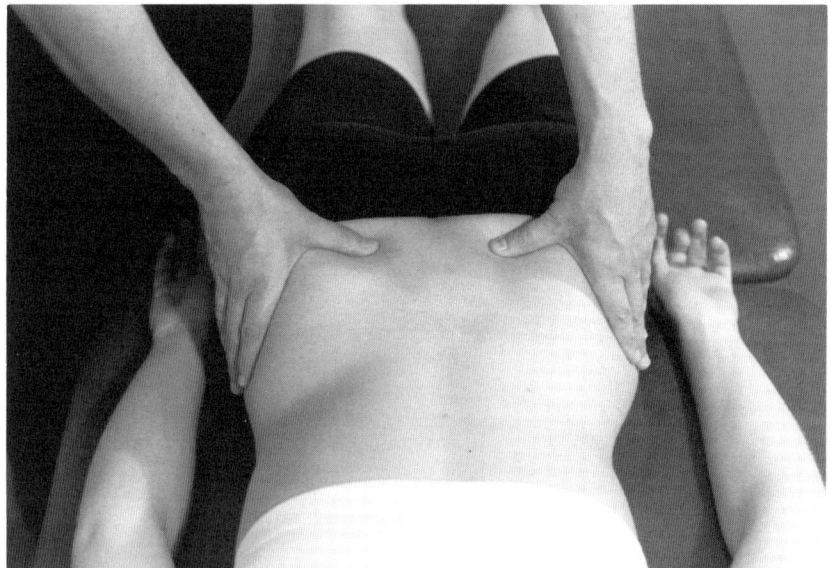

NOTES:

_____

_____

_____

_____

_____

_____

_____

POSITIONAL TESTS — INNOMINATE

Ischium

Patient: Prone.
Therapist: Standing at the patient's side.
Palpate: Initially, palpate the ischial tuberosity through the soft tissue at the gluteal fold with the heel of the hand. Then using the thumbs, palpate the most inferior aspect of the tuberosities. Compare the craniocaudal relationship of the two sides.

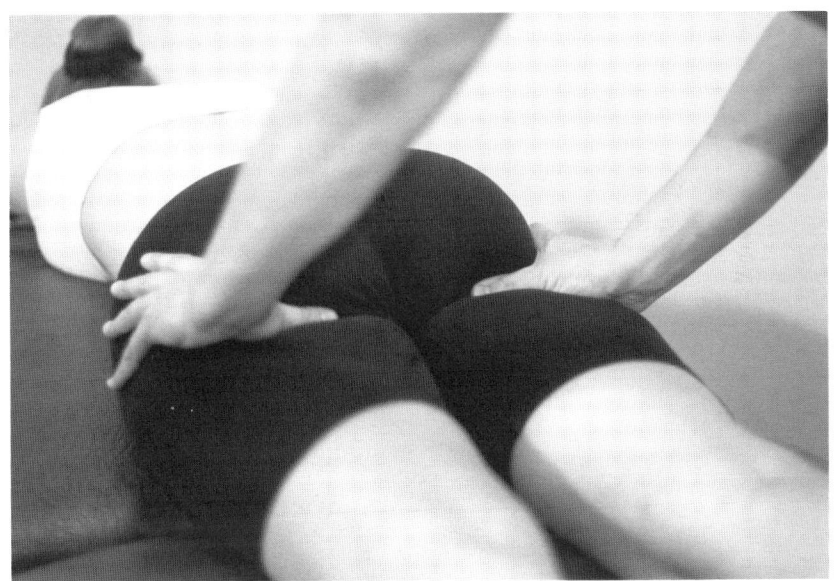

NOTES:

_____

_____

_____

_____

_____

_____

_____

_____

_____

_____

_____

POSITIONAL TESTS – SACRUM

Sacral Base – S1

Patient: Prone.
Therapist: Standing at the patient's side.
Palpate: With the thumbs, palpate the sacral base (S1) bilaterally medial to the inferior aspect of the PSIS's.
a) Note the dorsoventral relationship of the two sides relative to the coronal body plane. A dorsal left sacral base is suggestive of a left rotated sacral base.
b) Compare the position of the sacral base to the L5 vertebra. There is considerable asymmetry of the sacrum and positional changes should be correlated with mobility findings to determine the significance.
c) The left and right sacral sulcus depths can help in determining the position of the sacrum between the innominate bones. The depth of the sacral sulcus is noted by palpating the distance from the sacral base to the posterior aspect of the PSIS.

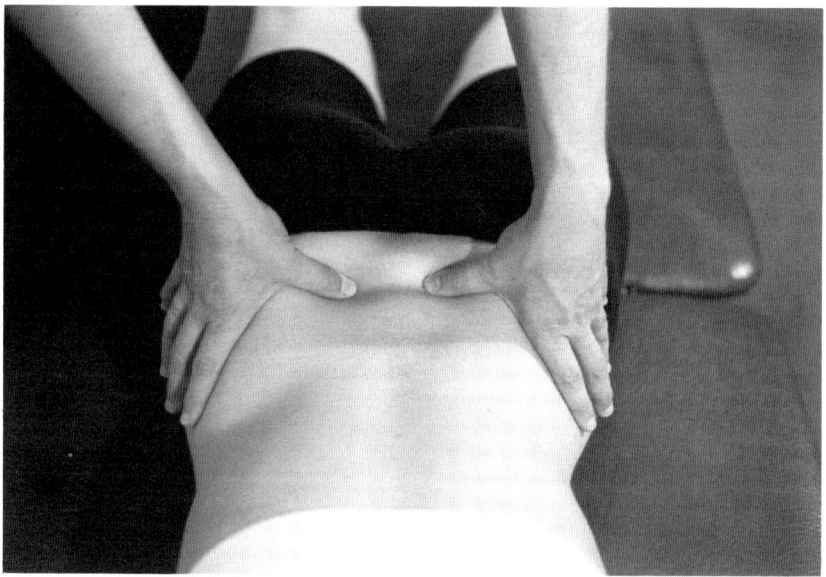

NOTES:

_____

_____

_____

_____

_____

POSITIONAL TESTS — SACRUM

S2, S3, S4

Patient: Prone.
Therapist: Standing at the patient's side.
Palpate: With the thumbs, palpate the sacrum medial to the PIIS's.
a) Note the dorsoventral relationship of the two sides relative to the coronal body plane. A dorsal left S2, S3, S4 is suggestive of a left rotation of the inferior aspect of the sacrum.
b) Compare the position of the inferior aspect of the sacrum to the sacral base. There is considerable asymmetry of the sacrum and positional changes should be correlated with mobility findings to determine the significance.

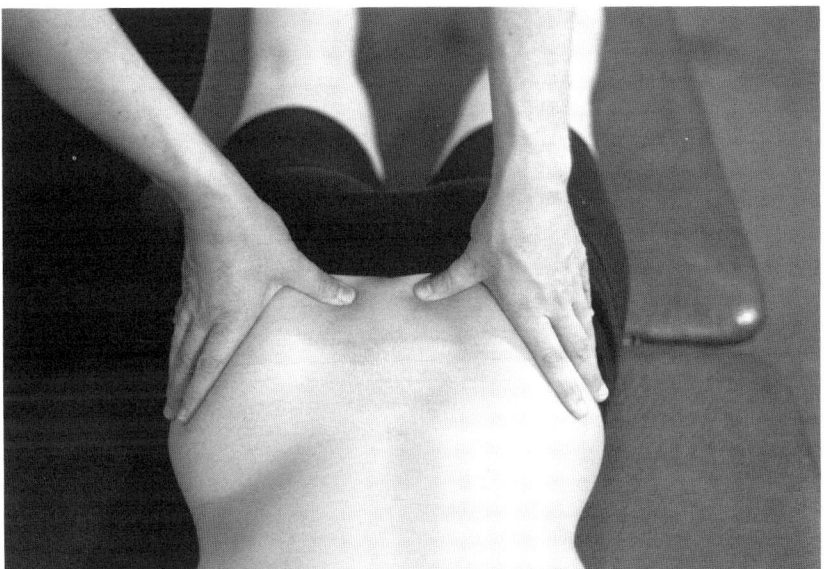

NOTES:

_____

_____

_____

_____

_____

_____

_____

_____

POSITIONAL TESTS — SACRUM

Inferior lateral angle – S5

Patient: Prone.
Therapist: Standing at the patient's side.
Palpate: With the index finger, palpate the median sacral crest inferiorly to reach the sacral hiatus. From this position, palpate inferolaterally to reach the dorsal aspect of the inferior lateral angle of the sacrum. With the thumbs, note the dorsoventral relationship of the two sides relative to the coronal body plane. There is considerable asymmetry of the sacrum and positional changes should be correlated with mobility findings to determine the significance.

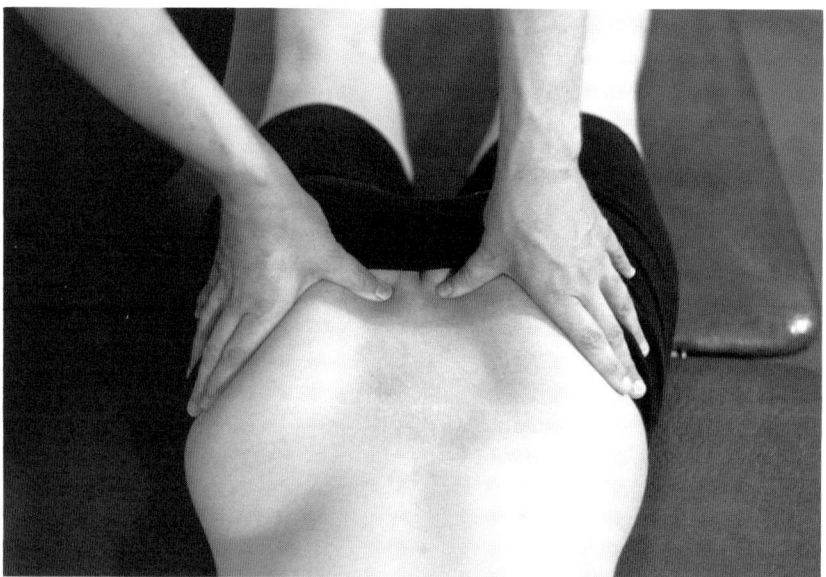

NOTES:

_____

_____

_____

_____

_____

_____

_____

_____

_____

ACTIVE MOBILITY TESTS OF OSTEOKINEMATIC FUNCTION

Forward bending

Patient: Standing, feet directly under the hips, with even distribution of body weight through both lower limbs.

Therapist: Standing behind the patient.

Palpate: With the thumbs, palpate the inferior aspect of the posterior superior iliac spines (PSIS's).

Test: Instruct the patient to forward bend keeping the knees extended. Observe and palpate the symmetry of the motion of both PSIS's, which should move equally in a superior direction. This test is not a sacroiliac articular mobility test, but rather a test of lower quadrant function in forward bending. The mobility of the pelvic girdle in this test is influenced by:

1. the stability of the lumbar spine and the pelvic girdle under body weight
2. the mobility of the lumbar, sacroiliac and hip joints
3. the muscle tension in the posterior aspect of the trunk, pelvis and lower limbs
4. the functional length of the lower extremities
5. the axis around which the motion occurs.

Asymmetry is indicative of dysfunction in the lower quadrant. The test may be repeated in sitting to eliminate the influence of some of the lower quadrant factors.

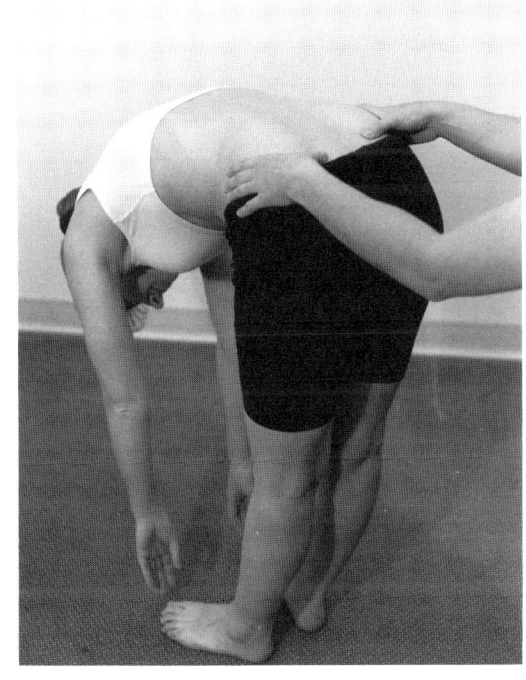

ACTIVE MOBILITY TESTS OF OSTEOKINEMATIC FUNCTION

Backward bending

Patient:	Standing, feet directly under the hips, even distribution of body weight through both lower limbs.
Therapist:	Standing behind the patient.
Palpate:	With the thumbs, palpate the inferior aspect of the posterior superior iliac spines (PSIS's).
Test:	Instruct the patient to backward bend. Observe and palpate the symmetry of the motion of both PSIS's, which should move equally in an inferior direction. This test is not a sacroiliac articular mobility test, but rather a test of lower quadrant function in backward bending. (See further notes in forward bending).

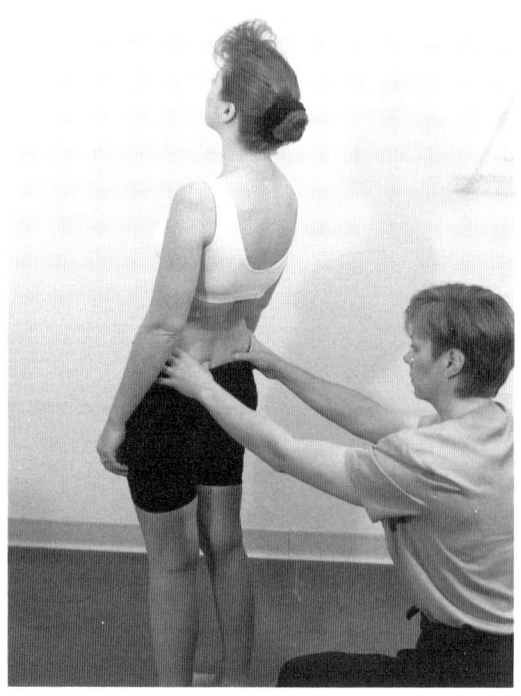

NOTES:

_____

_____

_____

_____

_____

_____

_____

ACTIVE MOBILITY TESTS OF OSTEOKINEMATIC FUNCTION

Posterior rotation – kinetic test - PSIS

Patient: Standing, feet directly under the hips, with even distribution of body weight through both lower limbs.

Therapist: Standing behind the patient.

Palpate: With one thumb, palpate the inferior aspect of the posterior superior iliac spine (PSIS). With the other thumb, palpate the sacral base lateral to the median sacral crest directly parallel to the opposite thumb.

Test: Instruct the patient to flex the ipsilateral hip and knee to 90° and note the inferior displacement of the PSIS relative to the sacral base.

Addendum: The pelvis should remain in its initial coronal and horizontal plane. Note the patient's ability to balance on the weight bearing limb. In this posture, the line of gravity passes through the weight bearing sacroiliac joint to the arcuate line of the innominate bone and then to the hip joint. Sacroiliac joint dysfunction can potentially disrupt this weight transference and consequently alter the balance on that side.

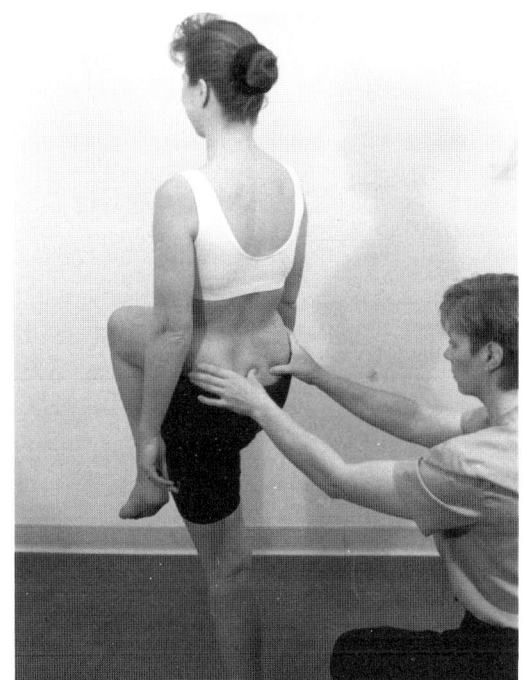

NOTES:

_____

_____

_____

ACTIVE MOBILITY TESTS OF OSTEOKINEMATIC FUNCTION

Posterior rotation – kinetic test – PIIS

Patient:	Standing, feet directly under the hips, with even distribution of body weight through both lower limbs.
Therapist:	Standing behind the patient.
Palpate:	With one thumb, palpate the posterior inferior iliac spine (PIIS). With the other thumb, palpate the sacrum directly parallel to this (S3).
Test:	Instruct the patient to flex the ipsilateral hip and knee to 90° and note the anterolateral displacement of the PIIS relative to the sacrum.

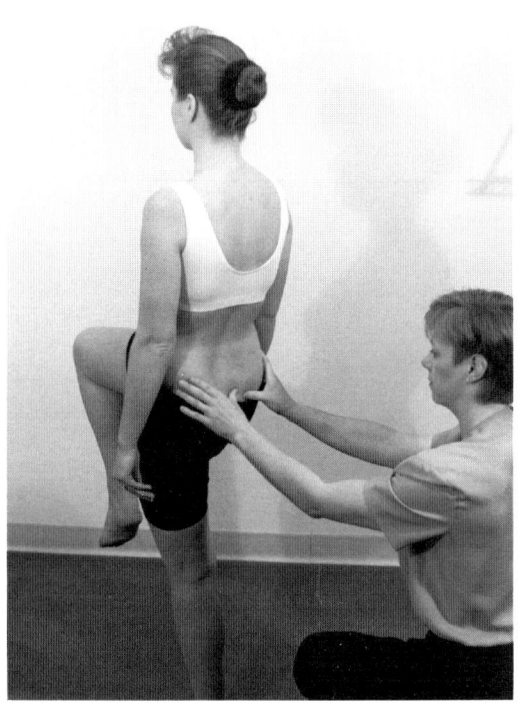

NOTES:

_____

_____

_____

_____

_____

_____

_____

_____

_____

ACTIVE MOBILITY TESTS OF OSTEOKINEMATIC FUNCTION

Anterior rotation – kinetic test – PSIS

Patient:	Standing, feet directly under the hips, with even distribution of body weight through both lower limbs.
Therapist:	Standing behind the patient.
Palpate:	With one thumb, palpate the inferior aspect of the posterior superior iliac spine (PSIS). With the other thumb, palpate the sacral base lateral to the median sacral crest directly parallel with the opposite thumb.
Test:	Instruct the patient to extend the ipsilateral hip with the knee extended and note the superior displacement of the PSIS relative to the sacral base.

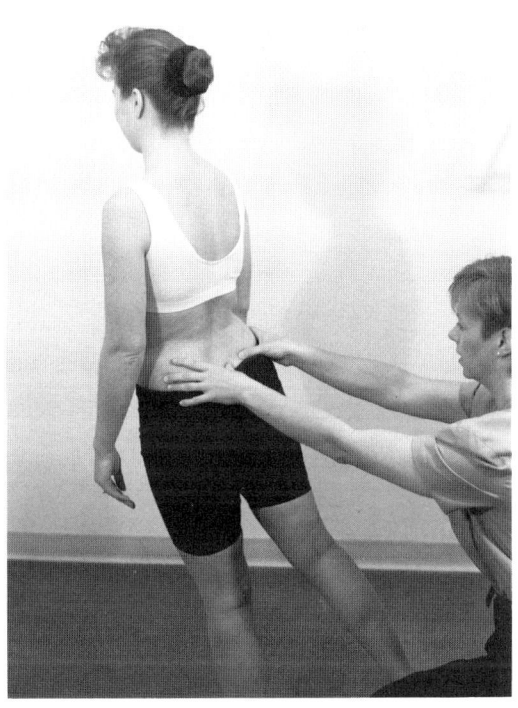

NOTES:

_____

_____

_____

_____

_____

_____

_____

ACTIVE MOBILITY TESTS OF OSTEOKINEMATIC FUNCTION

Anterior rotation – kinetic test – PIIS

Patient:	Standing, feet directly under the hips, with even distribution of body weight through both lower limbs.
Therapist:	Standing beside the patient.
Palpate:	With one thumb, palpate the posterior inferior iliac spine (PIIS). With the other thumb, palpate the sacrum directly parallel to this (S3).
Test:	Instruct the patient to extend the ipsilateral hip with the knee extended and note the posteromedial displacement of the PIIS relative to the sacrum.

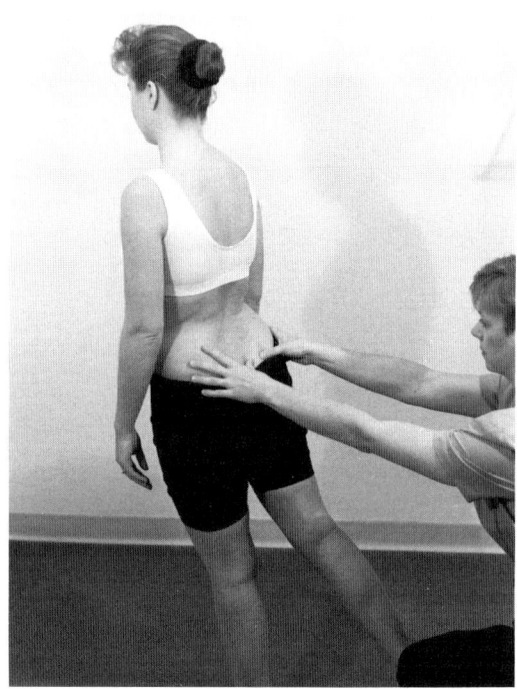

NOTES:

_____

_____

_____

_____

_____

_____

_____

_____

PASSIVE MOBILITY TESTS OF ARTHROKINEMATIC FUNCTION

Inferoposterior glide – sacroiliac joint

Patient: Supine, with the knees and hips flexed.

Therapist: Standing at the patient's side.

Palpate: With the long and ring finger of one hand, palpate the sacral sulcus just medial to the PSIS. With the index finger of the same hand, palpate the lumbosacral junction. The long and ring finger monitor motion between the innominate bone and the sacrum while the index finger notes any movement between the pelvic girdle and the L5 vertebra. With the heel of the other hand, palpate the ipsilateral ASIS and the iliac crest.

Test: Apply an anterior rotation force to the innominate bone to produce an inferoposterior glide at the sacroiliac joint. Note the quantity, direction of ease and the end feel of motion. This glide is also associated with counternutation of the sacrum. The glide is named as though the innominate were the moving bone. The end of the range of motion is reached when the pelvic girdle is felt to rotate as a unit beneath the L5 vertebra.

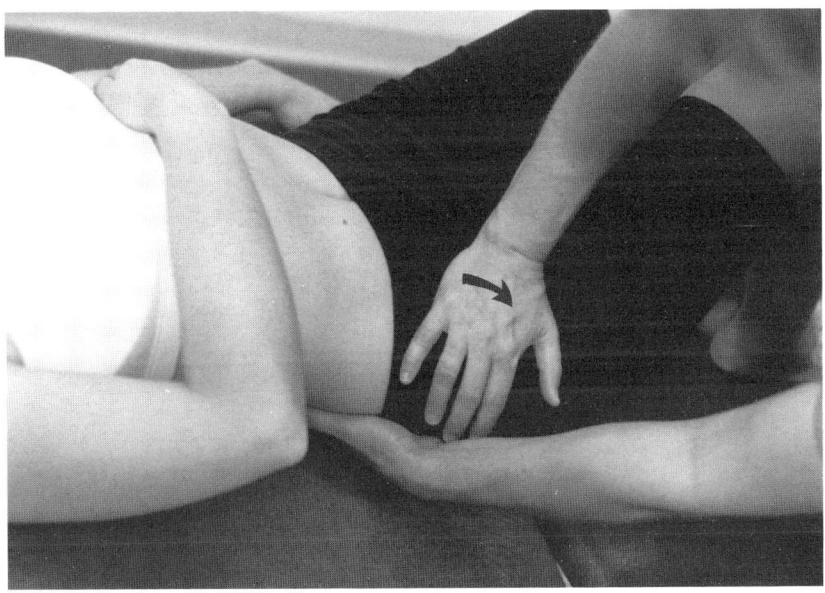

NOTES:

_____

_____

_____

_____

PASSIVE MOBILITY TESTS OF ARTHROKINEMATIC FUNCTION

Superoanterior glide – sacroiliac joint

Patient: Supine, with the knees and hips flexed.

Therapist: Standing at the patient's side.

Palpate: With the long and ring finger of one hand, palpate the sacral sulcus just medial to the PSIS. With the index finger of the same hand, palpate the lumbosacral junction. The long and ring finger monitor motion between the innominate bone and the sacrum while the index finger notes any movement between the pelvic girdle and the L5 vertebra. With the heel of the other hand, palpate the ipsilateral ASIS and the iliac crest.

Test: Apply a posterior rotation force to the innominate bone to produce a superoanterior glide at the sacroiliac joint. Note the quantity, direction of ease and the end feel of motion. This glide is also associated with nutation of the sacrum. The glide is named as though the innominate were the moving bone. The end of the range of motion is reached when the pelvic girdle is felt to rotate as a unit beneath the L5 vertebra.

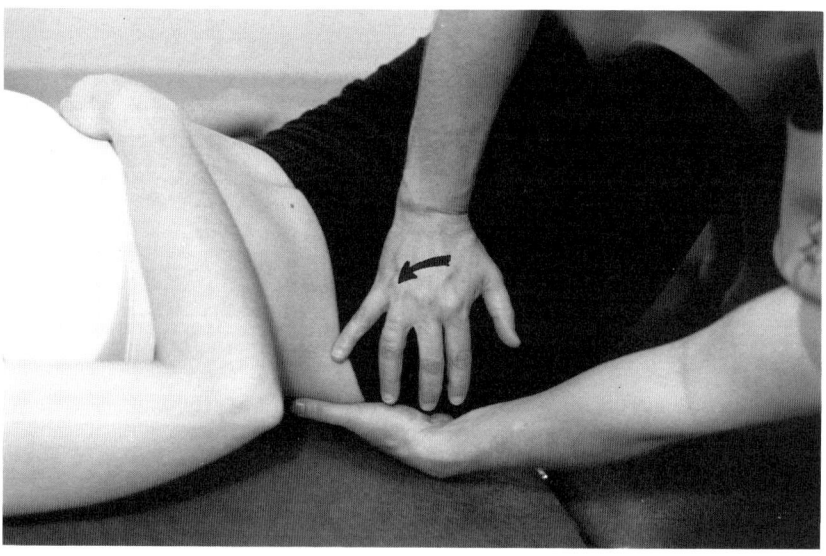

NOTES:

_____

_____

_____

_____

_____

PASSIVE STABILITY TESTS OF ARTHROKINETIC FUNCTION

Distraction (anterior)/Compression (posterior)

Patient:	Supine.
Therapist:	Standing at the patient's side.
Palpate:	With crossed arms, palpate the medial aspect of the ASIS's with the heels of the hands.
Test:	Apply a slow, steady force dorsolaterally (arrows) through the ASIS's thus stressing the ventral sacroiliac ligament and indirectly, the transverse pubic ligament. This force distracts the sacroiliac joints anteriorly and compresses them posteriorly. Maintain this force for 20 seconds and note any symptoms.

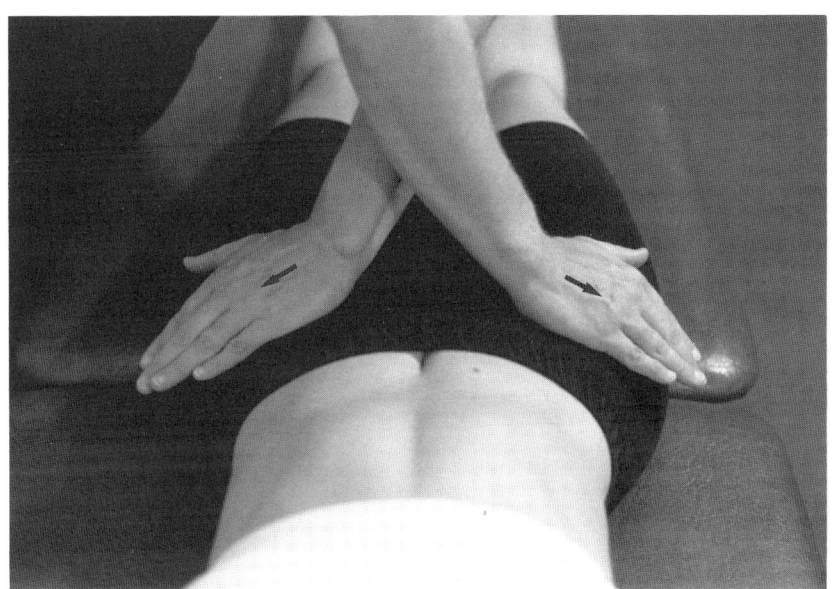

NOTES: _____

_____

_____

_____

_____

_____

_____

_____

_____

_____

PASSIVE STABILITY TESTS OF ARTHROKINETIC FUNCTION

Compression (anterior)/Distraction (posterior)

Patient:	Side lying, both hips and knees flexed.
Therapist:	Standing behind the patient.
Palpate:	With the heel of the hand, palpate the anterolateral aspect of the iliac crest. Reinforce this hand with the other.
Test:	Apply a slow, steady pressure towards the table (arrow) through the ventral aspect of the ilium. This force distracts the sacroiliac joints posteriorly and compresses them anteriorly. Maintain this force for 20 seconds and note any symptoms.

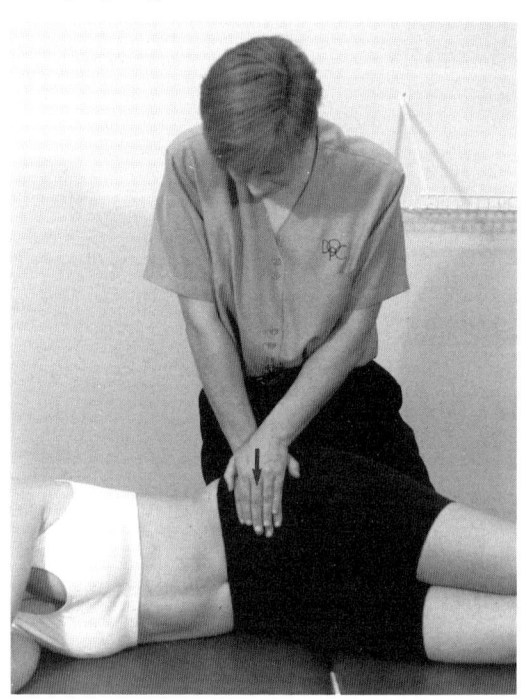

NOTES:

_____

_____

_____

_____

_____

_____

_____

_____

PASSIVE STABILITY TESTS OF ARTHROKINETIC FUNCTION

Posterior translation (innominate on sacrum) – supine

Patient:	Supine, with the knees and hips flexed.
Therapist:	Standing at the patient's side.
Palpate:	With the long and ring finger of one hand, palpate the sacral sulcus just medial to the PSIS. With the index finger of the same hand, palpate the lumbosacral junction. The long and ring finger monitor translation between the innominate bone and the sacrum while the index finger notes any movement between the pelvic girdle and the L5 vertebra. With the heel of the other hand, palpate the ipsilateral ASIS and the iliac crest.
Test:	Apply an anteroposterior force (arrow) to the ASIS and iliac crest and note the quantity and the end feel of motion as well as the reproduction of any symptoms. Sustain the force until the end feel is perceived. The end of the range of motion is reached when the pelvic girdle is felt to rotate as a unit beneath the L5 vertebra.

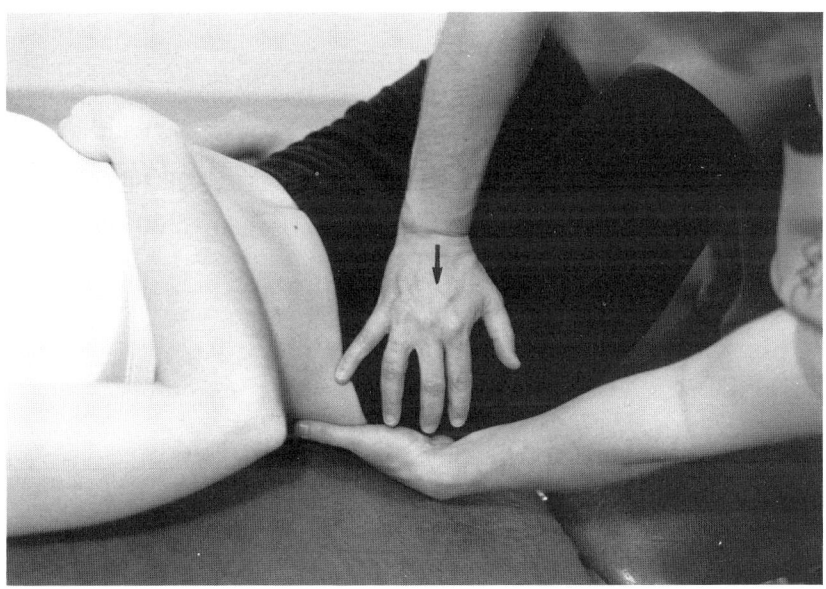

NOTES:

_____

_____

_____

_____

_____

PASSIVE STABILITY TESTS OF ARTHROKINETIC FUNCTION

Posterior translation (innominate on sacrum) – prone

Patient:	Prone.
Therapist:	Standing at the patient's side.
Palpate:	With one hand, palpate and fix the ASIS and iliac crest of the innominate bone. With the heel of the other hand, palpate the sacrum on the ipsilateral side.
Test:	Fix the innominate bone and apply a posteroanterior force (arrow) to the sacrum. Sustain the force until the end feel is perceived. Note the quantity and the end feel of motion as well as the reproduction of any symptoms.

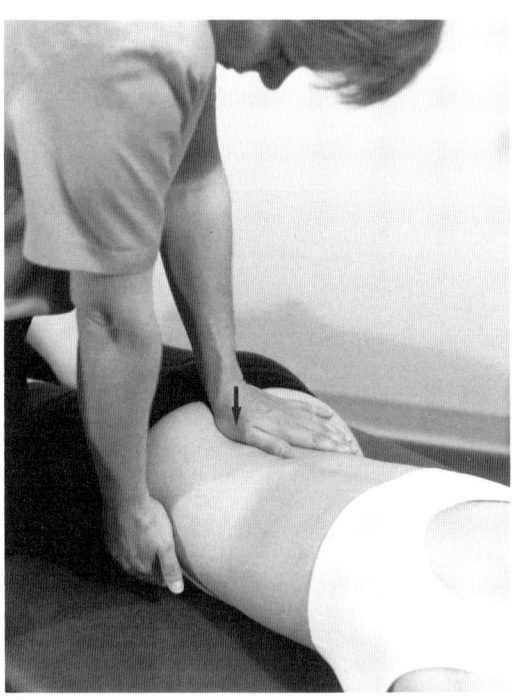

NOTES: _____

_____

_____

_____

_____

_____

_____

_____

PASSIVE STABILITY TESTS OF ARTHROKINETIC FUNCTION

Anterior translation (innominate on sacrum)

Patient: Prone.

Therapist: Standing at the patient's side.

Palpate: With one hand, palpate the PSIS and iliac crest of the innominate bone. With the heel of the other hand, palpate the sacrum on the contralateral side.

Test: Fix the sacrum and apply a posteroanterior force (arrow) to the innominate bone. Sustain the force until the end feel is perceived and note the quantity and the end feel of motion as well as the reproduction of any symptoms.

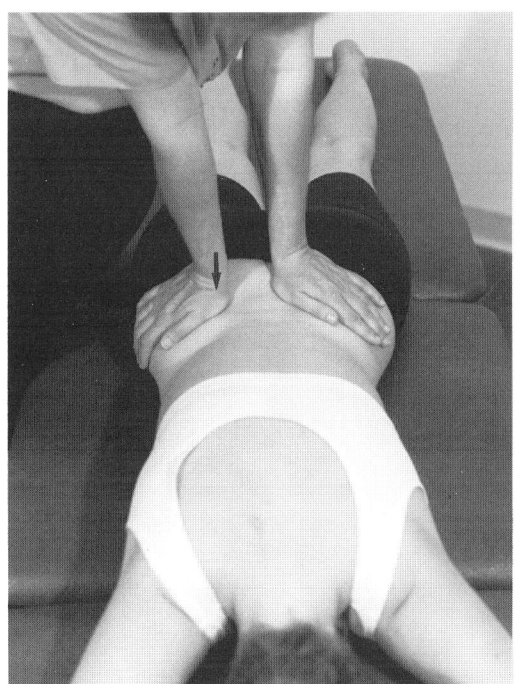

NOTES:

_____

_____

_____

_____

_____

_____

_____

_____

_____

PASSIVE STABILITY TESTS OF ARTHROKINETIC FUNCTION

Inferior translation (innominate on sacrum)

Patient: Prone.
Therapist: Standing at the patient's side.
Palpate: With one hand, palpate the iliac crest of the innominate bone. With the other hand, palpate the inferolateral aspect of the sacrum.
Test: Fix the sacrum and apply a superoinferior force to the innominate. Sustain the force until the end feel is perceived. Note the quantity and the end feel of motion as well as the reproduction of any symptoms.

Superior translation (innominate on sacrum)

Patient: Prone.
Therapist: Standing at the patient's side.
Palpate: With one hand, palpate and fix the sacral base. With the other hand, palpate the ischial tuberosity.
Test: Fix the sacrum and apply an inferosuperior force to the ischial tuberosity. Sustain the force until the end feel is perceived. Note the quantity and the end feel of motion as well as the reproduction of any symptoms.

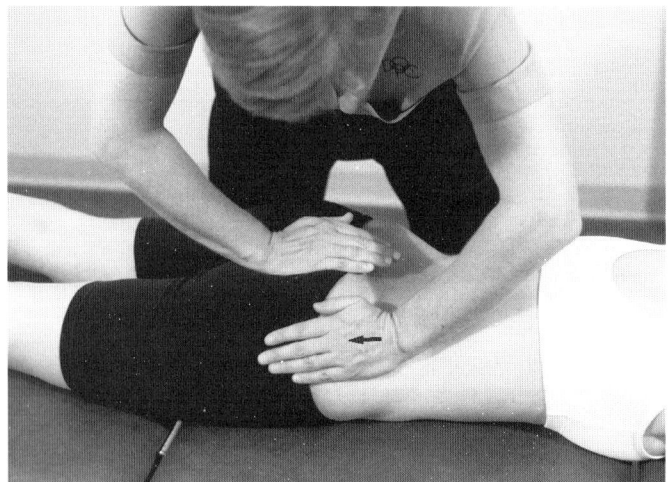 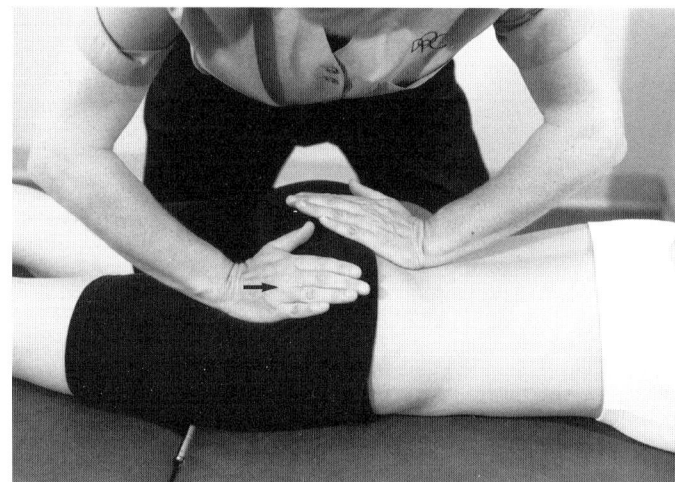

NOTES:

_____

_____

_____

_____

_____

PASSIVE STABILITY TESTS OF ARTHROKINETIC FUNCTION

Superoinferior translation (innominate on sacrum)

Patient:	Supine, with one hip and knee flexed and the distal end of the opposite femur resting over the therapist's knee.
Therapist:	Standing at the patient's side with one knee on the table.
Palpate:	With the long and ring finger of one hand, palpate the sacral sulcus just medial to the PSIS. With the index finger of the same hand, palpate the lumbosacral junction. The long and ring finger monitor translation between the innominate bone and the sacrum while the index finger notes any movement between the pelvic girdle and the L5 vertebra. With the other hand, palpate the distal end of the femur which is resting on the therapist's knee.
Test:	Apply an inferosuperior force then a superoinferior force to the distal end of the femur and note the quantity and the end feel of motion as well as the reproduction of any symptoms. Sustain the force until the end feel is perceived. The end of the range of motion is reached when the pelvic girdle is felt to sideflex as a unit beneath the L5 vertebra.

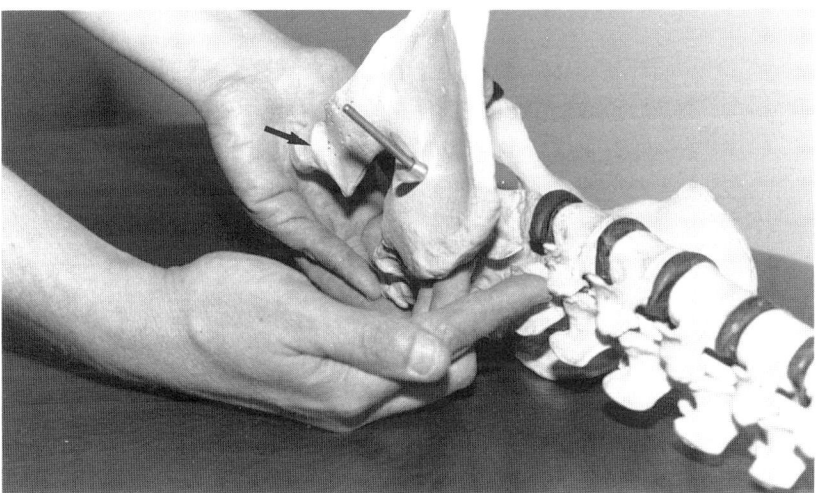

NOTES:

_____

_____

_____

_____

_____

_____

_____

PASSIVE STABILITY TESTS OF ARTHROKINETIC FUNCTION

Superoinferior translation – pubic symphysis

Patient: Supine.
Therapist: Standing at the patient's side.
Palpate: With the heel of one hand, palpate the superior aspect of the superior ramus of one pubic bone. With the heel of the other hand, palpate the inferior aspect of the superior ramus of the opposite pubic bone.
Test: Fix one pubic bone and apply a slow, steady inferosuperior force to the other and note the quantity and the end feel of motion as well as the reproduction of any symptoms. Switch hands and repeat the test such that each side is stressed superiorly and inferiorly.

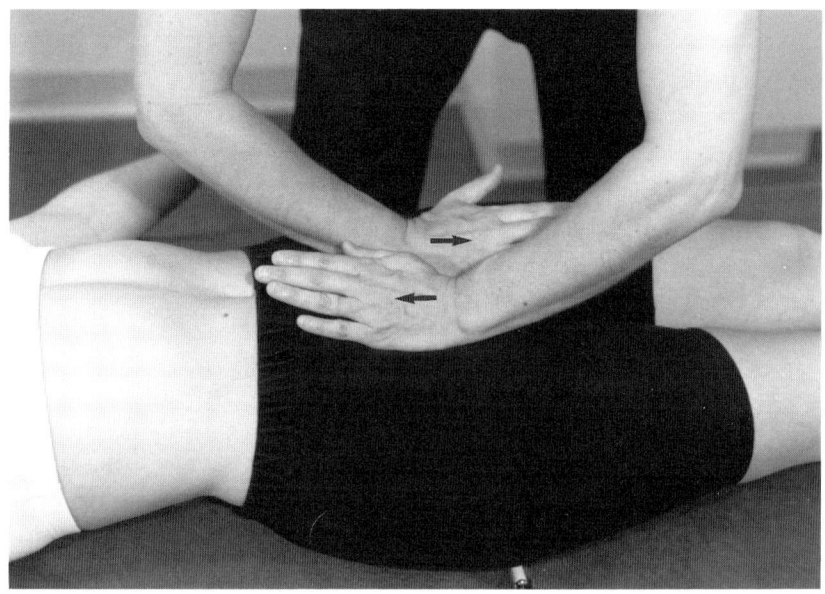

NOTES:

_____

_____

_____

_____

_____

_____

_____

_____

PASSIVE STABILITY TESTS OF ARTHROKINETIC FUNCTION

Sacrotuberous ligament tension

Patient:	Prone.
Therapist:	Standing at the patient's side.
Palpate & Test:	With the heel of the hands, locate the ischial tuberosities through the soft tissue at the gluteal folds. Then with the thumbs, palpate the inferomedial aspect of the ischial tuberosities. From this point, slide superolaterally to palpate the sacrotuberous ligament. Compare the relative tension between the left and the right side.

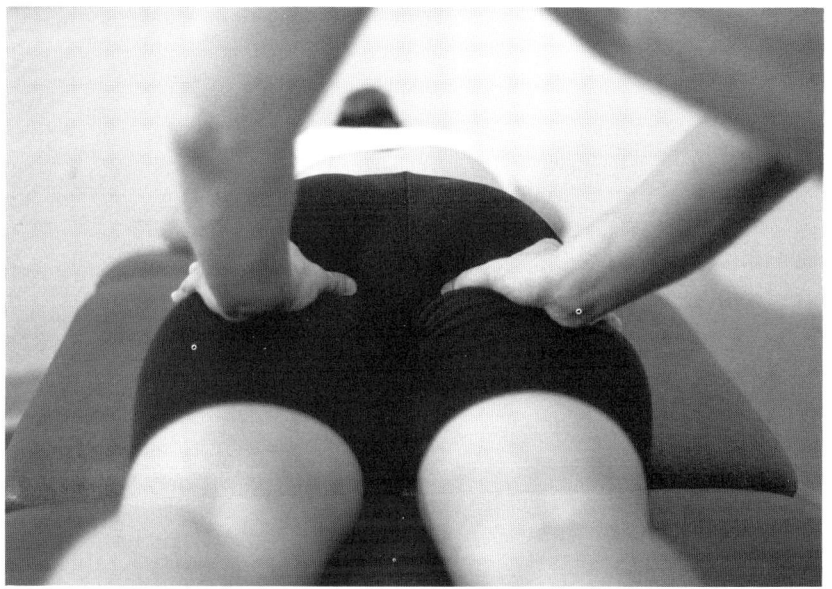

NOTES:

_____

_____

_____

_____

_____

_____

_____

_____

_____

_____

_____

PASSIVE STABILITY TESTS OF ARTHROKINETIC FUNCTION

Sacrotuberous/Interosseous ligaments

Patient: Prone.
Therapist: Standing at the patient's side.
Palpate: With the heel of one hand, palpate the sacral base in the midline. Reinforce this hand with the other.
Test: Apply an anterior force bilaterally to the sacral base thus forcing the sacrum to nutate. Maintain this force for 20 seconds and note the reproduction of any symptoms.

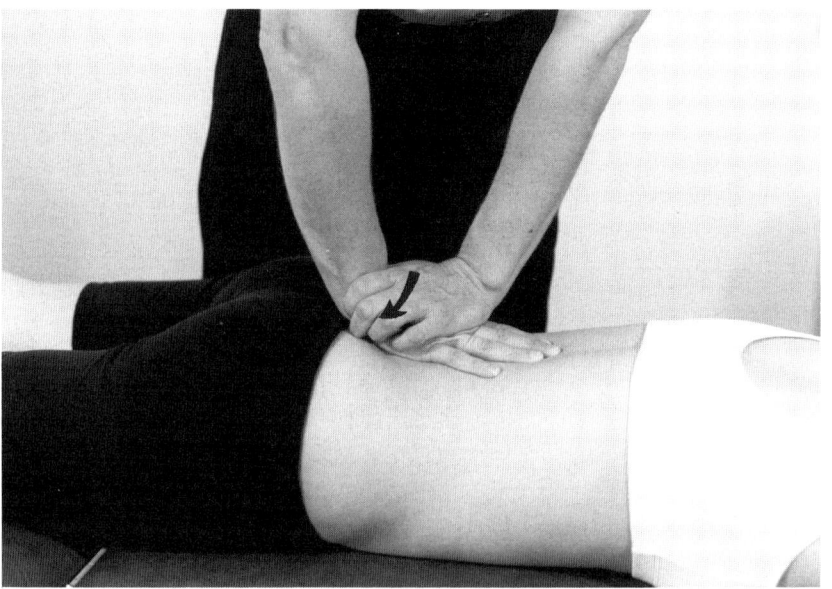

NOTES:

_____

_____

_____

_____

_____

_____

_____

_____

_____

_____

PASSIVE STABILITY TESTS OF ARTHROKINETIC FUNCTION

Long dorsal sacroiliac ligament

Patient: Prone.

Therapist: Standing at the patient's side.

Palpate: With one hand, palpate the inferior aspect of the sacrum in the midline. Reinforce this hand with the other.

Test: Apply an anterior force to the sacrum thus forcing the sacrum to counternutate. Maintain this force for 20 seconds and note the reproduction of any symptoms.

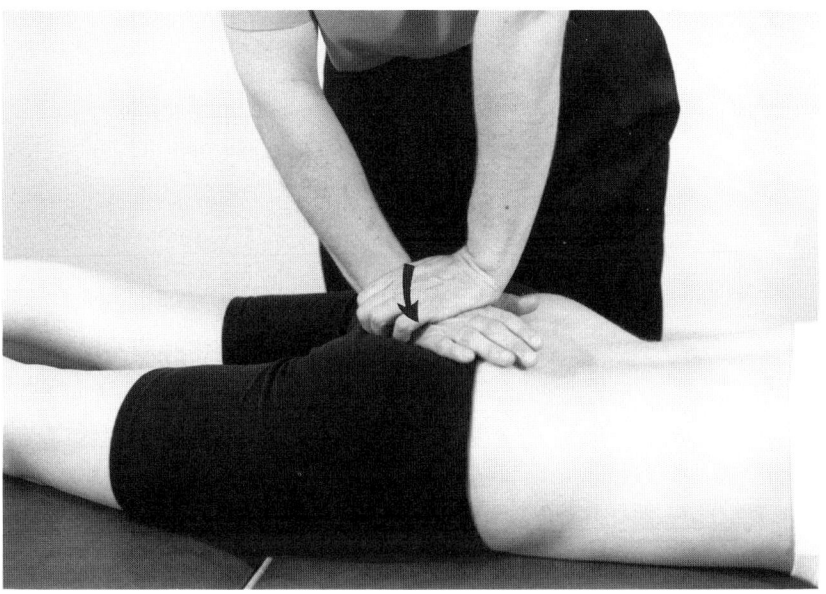

NOTES:

_____

_____

_____

_____

_____

_____

_____

_____

_____

_____

MOBILIZATION TECHNIQUES — INNOMINATE

Restriction of anterior rotation (inferoposterior glide – innominate on sacrum)

Patient: Supine, with the knees and hips flexed.

Therapist: Standing at the patient's side.

Palpate: With the long and ring finger of one hand, palpate the sacral sulcus just medial to the PSIS. With the index finger of the same hand, palpate the lumbosacral junction. The long and ring finger monitor motion between the innominate bone and the sacrum while the index finger notes any movement between the pelvic girdle and the L5 vertebra. With the heel of the other hand, palpate the ipsilateral ASIS and the iliac crest.

Mobilization: Apply a grade 2 to 4 anterior rotation force to the ASIS and iliac crest to produce an inferoposterior glide at the sacroiliac joint.

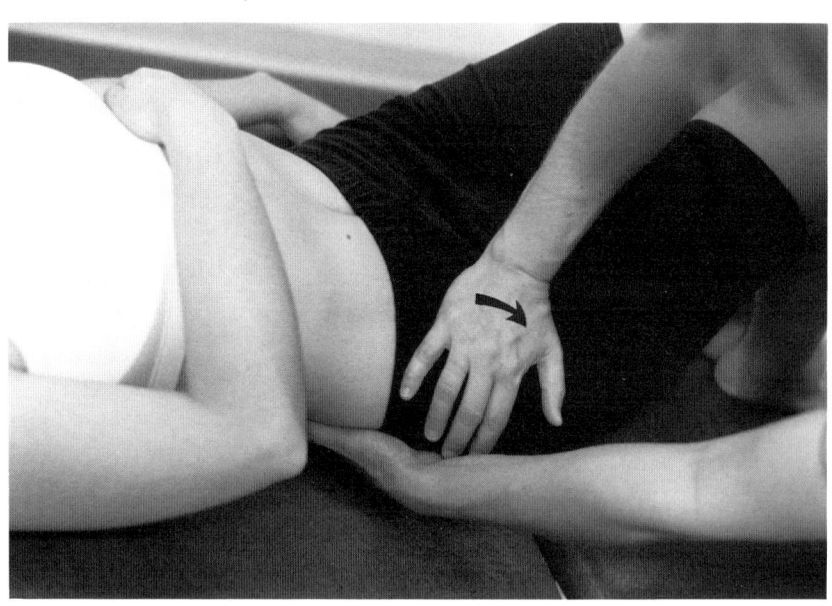

NOTES:

_____

_____

_____

_____

_____

_____

MOBILIZATION TECHNIQUES – INNOMINATE

Restriction of posterior rotation (superoanterior glide – innominate on sacrum)

Patient: Supine, with the knees and hips flexed.

Therapist: Standing at the patient's side.

Palpate: With the long and ring finger of one hand, palpate the sacral sulcus just medial to the PSIS. With the index finger of the same hand, palpate the lumbosacral junction. The long and ring finger monitor motion between the innominate bone and the sacrum while the index finger notes any movement between the pelvic girdle and the L5 vertebra. With the heel of the other hand, palpate the ipsilateral ASIS and the iliac crest.

Mobilization: Apply a grade 2 to 4 posterior rotation force to the ASIS and iliac crest to produce a superoanterior glide at the sacroiliac joint.

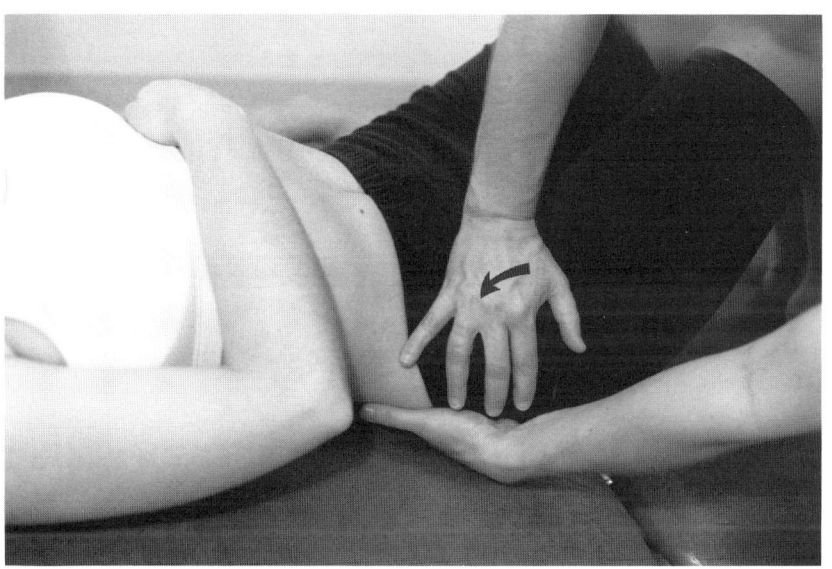

NOTES:

_____

_____

_____

_____

_____

_____

MOBILIZATION TECHNIQUES - INNOMINATE

Restriction of anterior rotation – left innominate – prone

Patient:	Prone.
Therapist:	Standing at the patient's side.
Palpate:	With one hand, support the anterior aspect of the thigh just above the left knee. With the heel of the other hand, palpate the PSIS of the left innominate bone.
Localization:	The motion barrier is localized by first extending the hip joint to the physiological limit. Further hip extension rotates the innominate anteriorly and this is continued until motion at the lumbosacral junction is perceived. The sacroiliac joint motion barrier has then been reached.
Mobilization:	**Active** – From this position, the patient is instructed to flex the hip against the therapist's resistance (arrow). This isometric contraction is held for up to 5 seconds following which the patient is instructed to completely relax. The new barrier to anterior rotation is localized by further extension of the hip joint. The mobilization is repeated 3 times and followed by a re-evaluation of osteokinematic, arthrokinematic and arthrokinetic function.

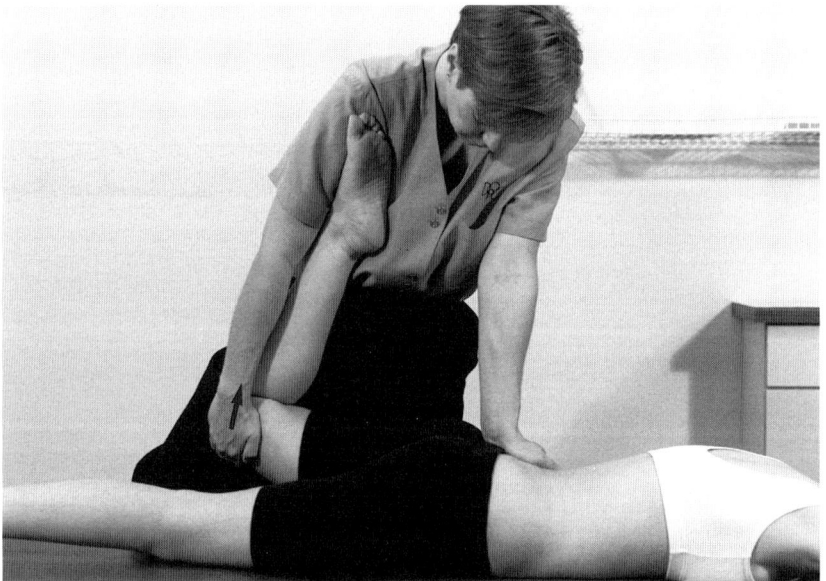

NOTES:

_____

_____

_____

_____

MOBILIZATION TECHNIQUES – INNOMINATE

Restriction of anterior rotation – left innominate – side lying

Patient: Right side lying, right hip and knee fully flexed and held by the patient.

Therapist: Standing behind the patient.

Palpate: With the thumb of one hand, palpate the sacral sulcus, allowing the rest of this hand to lie over the iliac crest. With the other hand, support the medial aspect of the left flexed knee. The lower leg rests on the therapist's forearm.

Localization: The motion barrier is localized by first extending the hip joint to the physiological limit. Further hip extension rotates the innominate anteriorly and this is continued until motion at the lumbosacral junction is perceived. The sacroiliac joint motion barrier has then been reached.

Mobilization: **Active** – From this position, the patient is instructed to flex the hip against the therapist's resistance (arrow). This isometric contraction is held for up to 5 seconds following which the patient is instructed to completely relax. The new barrier to anterior rotation is localized by further extension of the hip joint. The mobilization is repeated 3 times and followed by a re-evaluation of osteokinematic, arthrokinematic and arthrokinetic function.

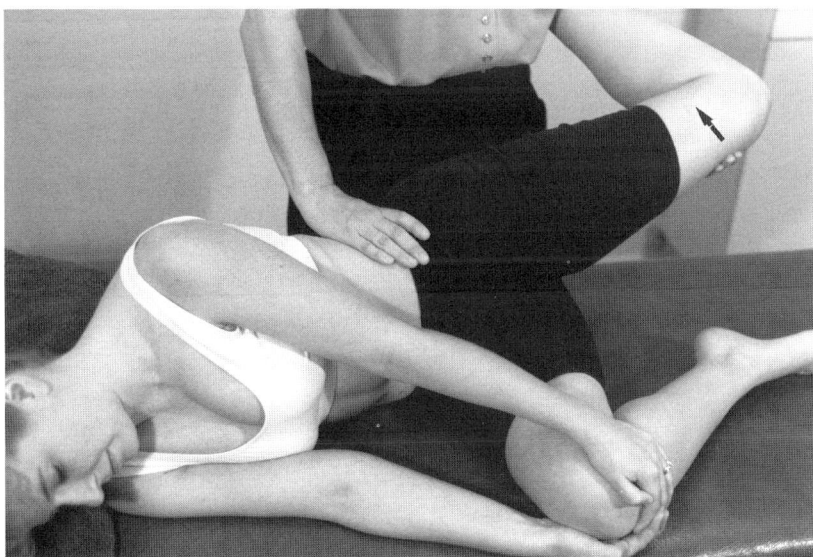

NOTES:

_____

_____

_____

MOBILIZATION TECHNIQUES – INNOMINATE

Restriction of posterior rotation – right innominate

Patient: Supine, hip and knee flexed.

Therapist: Standing at the patient's side.

Palpate: With one hand, cup the right ischial tuberosity. With the index and long fingers of the other hand, palpate the lumbosacral junction and the sacral sulcus.

Localization: The motion barrier is localized by first flexing the hip joint to the limit. Further hip flexion rotates the innominate posteriorly and this is continued until motion at the lumbosacral junction is perceived. The sacroiliac joint motion barrier has then been reached.

Mobilization: **Active** – From this position, the patient is instructed to extend the hip against the resistance provided by the therapist's shoulder (arrow). This isometric contraction is held for up to 5 seconds following which the patient is instructed to completely relax. The new barrier to posterior rotation is localized by further flexion of the hip joint. The mobilization is repeated 3 times and followed by a re-evaluation of osteokinematic, arthrokinematic and arthrokinetic function.

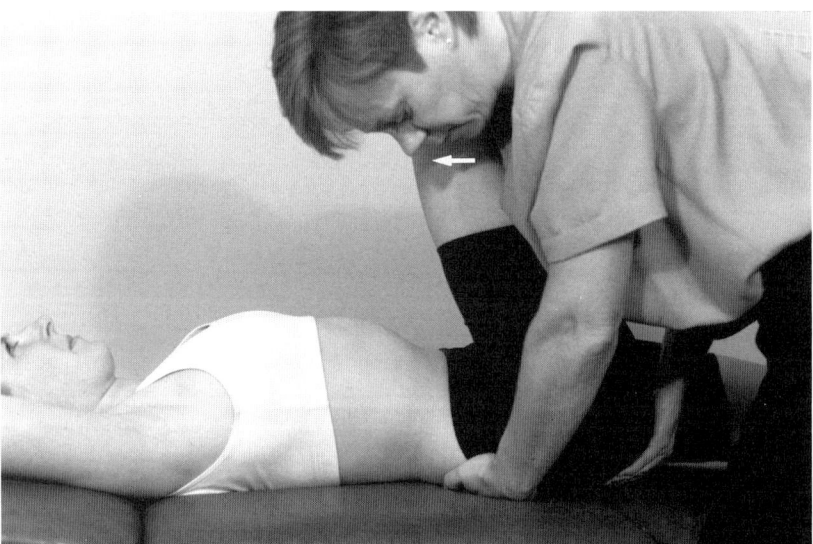

NOTES:

_____

_____

_____

_____

MOBILIZATION TECHNIQUES — INNOMINATE

Restriction of external rotation

Patient: Supine, hip and knee on the side of the lesion flexed.

Therapist: Standing at the patient's side.

Palpate: With one hand, palpate the ASIS and the iliac crest of the opposite innominate. With the other hand, palpate the medial aspect of the patient's flexed knee.

Localization: The motion barrier is localized by abducting and externally rotating the flexed hip joint to the physiological limit. Further abduction and external rotation of the hip joint is then gently applied, while fixing the contralateral innominate, thus using the flexed hip joint as a lever to rotate the innominate externally.

Mobilization: **Active** – From this position, the patient is instructed to adduct the hip against the therapist's resistance (arrow). This isometric contraction is held for up to 5 seconds following which the patient is instructed to completely relax. The new motion barrier is localized by further abduction and external rotation of the flexed hip joint. The mobilization is repeated 3 times and followed by a re-evaluation of osteokinematic, arthrokinematic and arthrokinetic function.

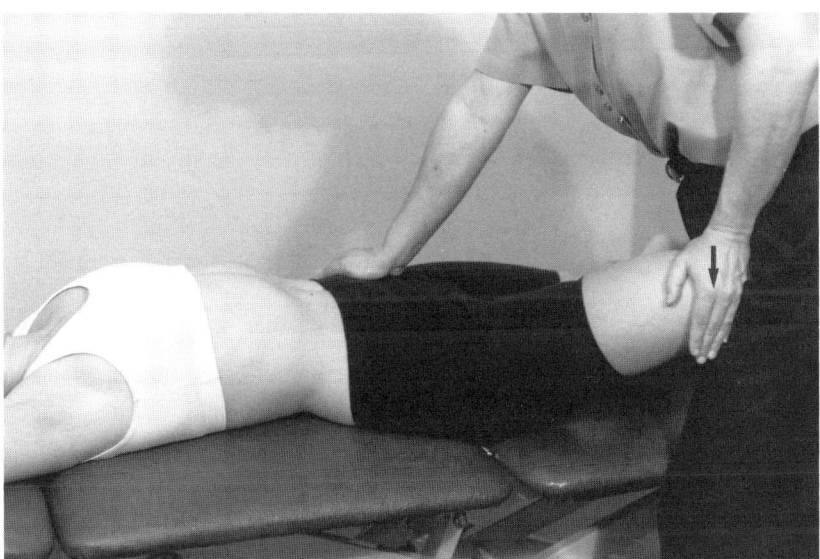

NOTES:

_____

_____

_____

MOBILIZATION TECHNIQUES — INNOMINATE

Restriction of internal rotation

Patient: Supine, hip and knee on the side of the lesion flexed.

Therapist: Standing at the patient's side.

Palpate: With the index and long finger of one hand, palpate the medial aspect of the PSIS on the side of the lesion. With the other hand, palpate the medial aspect of the flexed knee and cradle the lower leg against the shoulder.

Localization: The motion barrier is localized by internally rotating the innominate with the posterior hand (white arrow). Alternately, the barrier can be localized by adducting and internally rotating the flexed hip joint to the physiological limit. Further adduction and internal rotation of the hip joint is then gently applied thus using the fixed hip joint as a lever to rotate the innominate internally.

Mobilization: **Active** – From this position, the patient is instructed to abduct the hip against the resistance provided by the therapist's shoulder (arrow). This isometric contraction is held for up to 5 seconds following which the patient is instructed to completely relax. The new motion barrier is localized by further internal rotation of the innominate bone. The mobilization is repeated 3 times and followed by a re-evaluation of osteokinematic, arthrokinematic and arthrokinetic function.

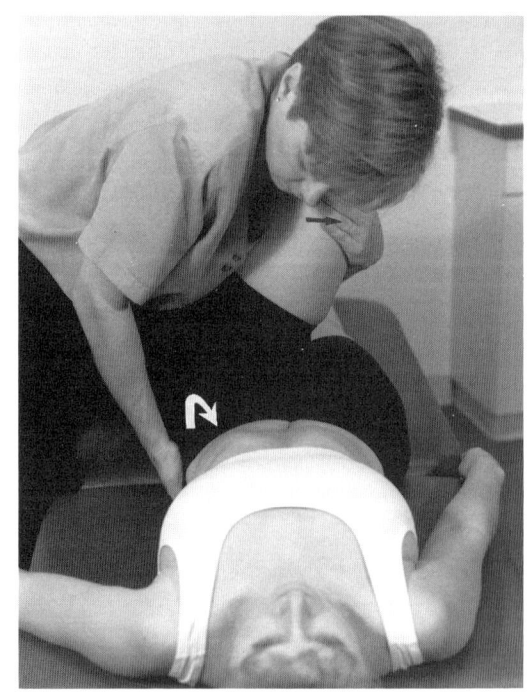

MOBILIZATION TECHNIQUES — SACRUM

Restriction of nutation (inferoposterior glide - sacrum on innominate)

Patient: Prone.
Therapist: Standing at the patient's side.
Palpate: With the thumb and index finger of one hand, palpate the sacral base bilaterally. Reinforce this hand with the other.
Mobilization: **Passive** – Apply a grade 2 to 4 nutation force to the sacral base to produce an inferoposterior glide at the sacroiliac joints.

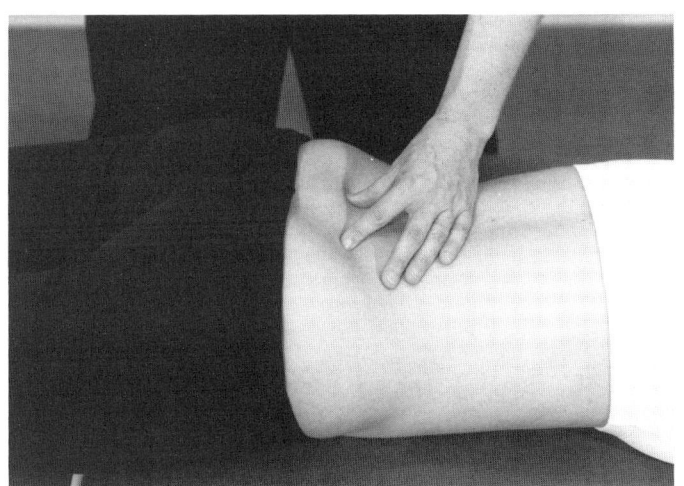 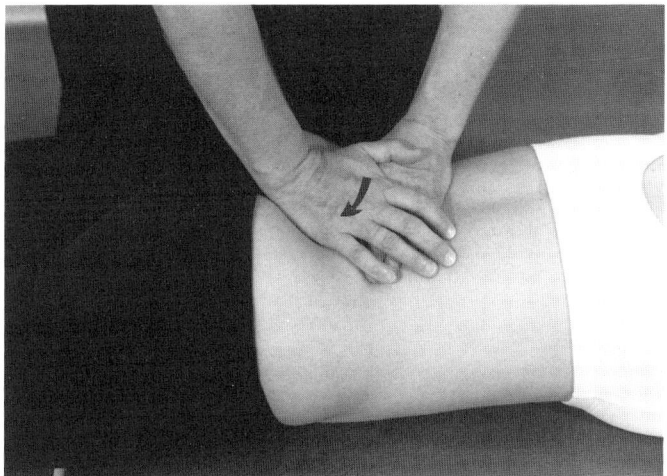

NOTES:

_____

_____

_____

_____

_____

_____

_____

_____

_____

_____

_____

MOBILIZATION TECHNIQUES – SACRUM

Restriction of counternutation (superoanterior glide – sacrum on innominate)

Patient: Prone.
Therapist: Standing at the patient's side.
Palpate: With the thumb and index finger of one hand, palpate the sacral base bilaterally. With the heel of the other hand, palpate the inferior aspect of the sacrum in the midline.
Mobilization: **Passive** – Apply a grade 2 to 4 counternutation force to the sacrum to produce a superoanterior glide at the sacroiliac joints.

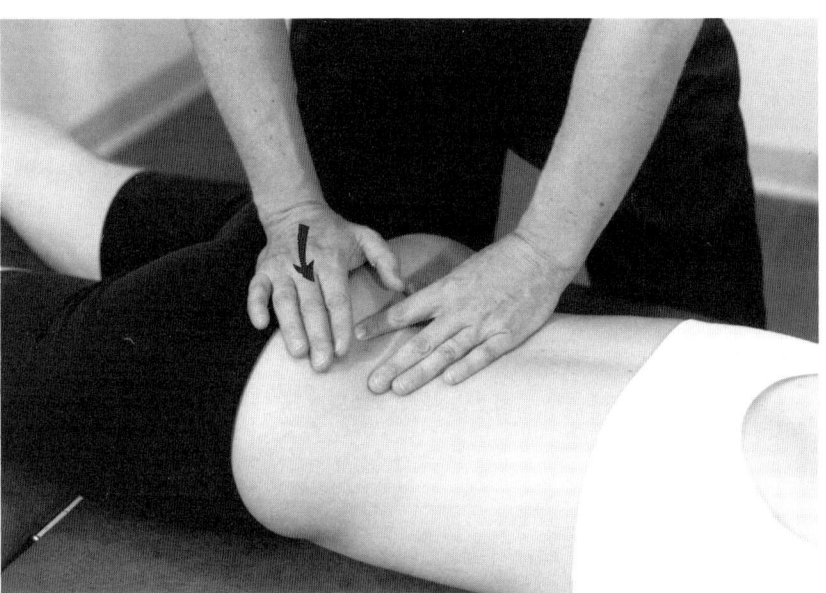

NOTES:

_____

_____

_____

_____

_____

_____

_____

_____

_____

_____

MOBILIZATION TECHNIQUES – SACRUM

Restriction of sacral counternutation – unilateral

Patient: Side lying, on the side to which the sacrum is rotated, with the trunk rotated towards the floor, the lower arm resting behind the back and the upper arm hanging over the edge of the table. The hips and knees are flexed.

Therapist: Standing facing the patient's flexed knees.

Palpate: With one hand, support the patient's feet allowing the femora to rest against the therapist's thigh. With the long finger of the other hand, palpate the interspinous space at L5-S1. With the index finger of this hand, palpate the dorsal aspect of the sacrum on the side which is restricted.

Localization: The L5-S1 joint is positioned in neutral. The knees are kept together and then lowered towards the floor just until the first resistance is met. From this point, the feet are lowered to the floor until the next resistance is met.

Mobilization: **Active** – From this position, the patient is instructed to prevent the feet from dropping towards the floor as the therapist lightly releases the support of the feet. This isometric contraction is held for up to 5 seconds following which the patient is instructed to completely relax. The mobilization is repeated 3 times and followed by a re-evaluation of osteokinematic, arthrokinematic and arthrokinetic function.

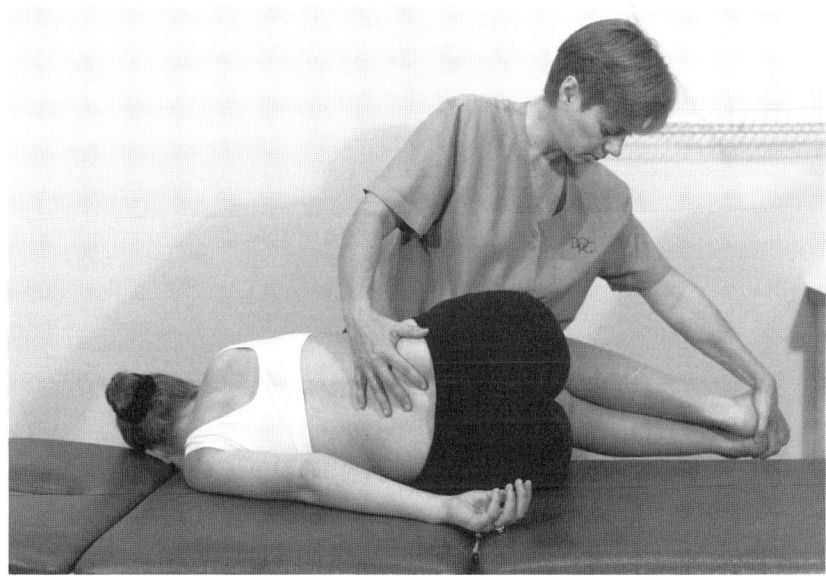

NOTES:

_____

_____

MOBILIZATION TECHNIQUES – SACRUM

Restriction of sacral nutation – unilateral

Patient: Side lying, on the side to which the sacrum is rotated, with the trunk in neutral, lower leg extended, upper hip and knee flexed.

Therapist: Standing facing the patient.

Localization: The L5-S1 joint is extended to the motion barrier. With the long finger, palpate the interspinous space at L5-S1. With the index finger of this hand, palpate the dorsal aspect of the sacrum on the side with is restricted.

Mobilization: Active – From this position, the therapist grasps the lower leg above the ankle and attempts to extend the hip (arrow). The iliopsoas muscle is recruited thus drawing the sacral base anteriorly. The antagonist, erector spinae, is released through reciprocal inhibition. The contraction is held for up to 5 seconds and followed by a period of complete relaxation. The technique is repeated 3 times and followed by a re-evaluation of osteokinematic, arthrokinematic and arthrokinetic function.

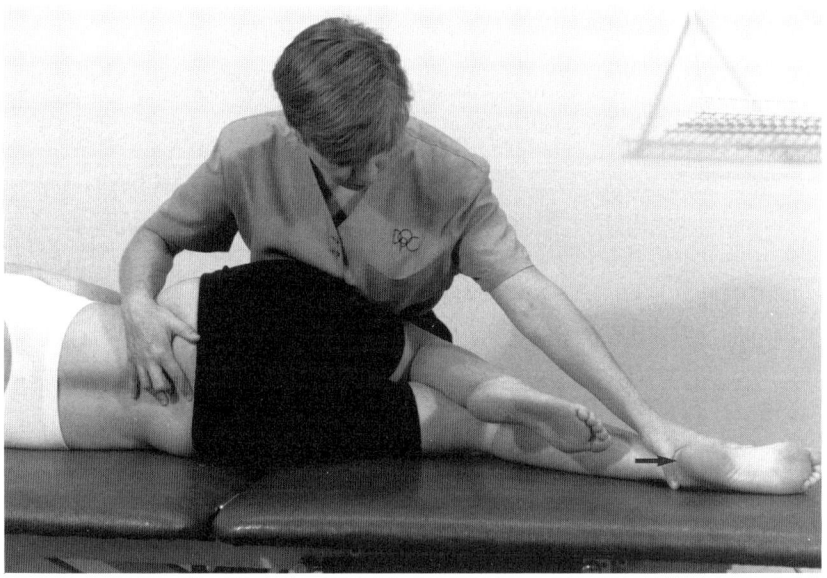

NOTES:
_____
_____
_____
_____
_____

MANIPULATION TECHNIQUES — INNOMINATE

Subluxation of the innominate – superior with anterior rotation

Patient: Prone.

Therapist: Standing at the end of the table facing the patient.

Palpate: With both hands, grasp the patient's lower leg, proximal to the talocrural joint, on the side being treated.

Manipulation: The motion barrier is reached by applying a longitudinal pull through the leg. A high velocity, low amplitude tug is applied through the leg to the sacroiliac joint. The technique is followed by a re-evaluation of osteokinematic, arthrokinematic and arthrokinetic function.

Addendum: A second therapist may assist by stabilizing the inferolateral aspect of the sacrum with the heel of one hand.

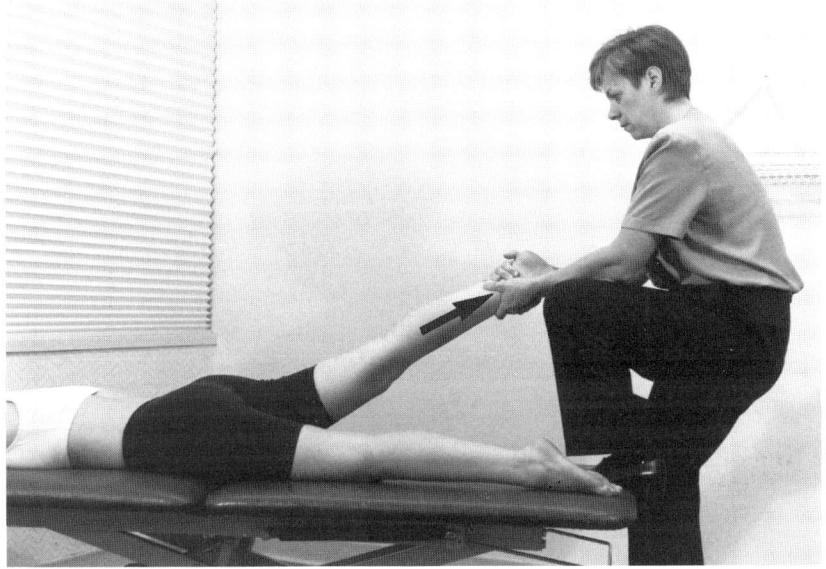

NOTES:

_____

_____

_____

_____

_____

_____

_____

_____

_____

MANIPULATION TECHNIQUES – INNOMINATE

Subluxation of the innominate – superior with posterior rotation

Patient: Supine.
Therapist: Standing at the end of the table facing the patient.
Palpate: With both hands, grasp the patient's lower leg, proximal to the talocrural joint, on the side being treated.
Manipulation: The motion barrier is reached by applying a longitudinal pull through the leg. A high velocity, low amplitude tug is applied through the leg to the sacroiliac joint. The technique is followed by a re-evaluation of osteokinematic, arthrokinematic and arthrokinetic function.

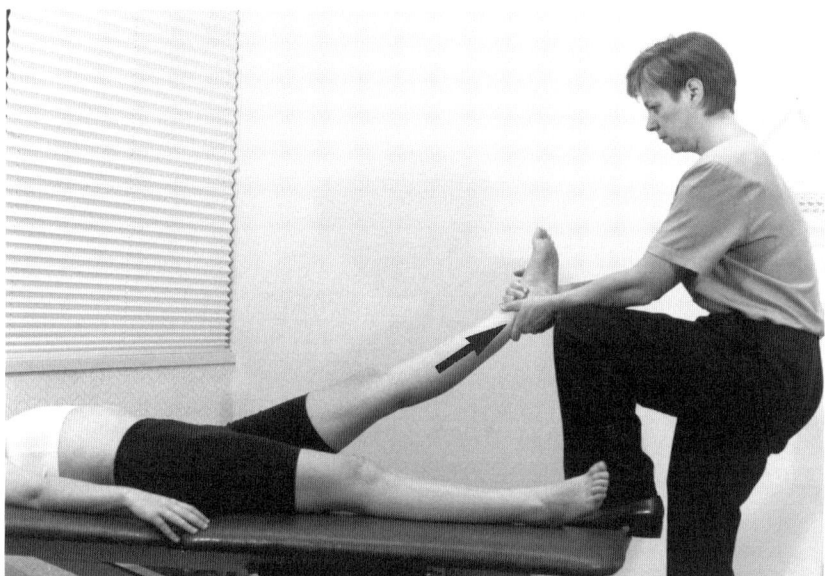

NOTES:

_____

_____

_____

_____

_____

_____

_____

_____

_____

_____

MANIPULATION TECHNIQUES – INNOMINATE

Subluxation of the innominate – right inferior

Patient: Supine, with the right hip and knee flexed and held by the patient.

Therapist: Standing at the end of the table facing the patient.

Palpate: With both hands, grasp the patient's extended left lower leg, proximal to the talocrural joint. Internally rotate the left leg until full internal rotation of the innominate is achieved. This locks the left sacroiliac joint.

Manipulation: The motion barrier of the right sacroiliac joint is reached by applying a longitudinal pull through the internally rotated left leg. The caudal force is transmitted to the right side of the sacrum through the locked left sacroiliac joint. This produces a relative superior glide of the right innominate. A high velocity, low amplitude tug is applied through the leg to the contralateral sacroiliac joint. The technique is followed by a re-evaluation of osteokinematic, arthrokinematic and arthrokinetic function.

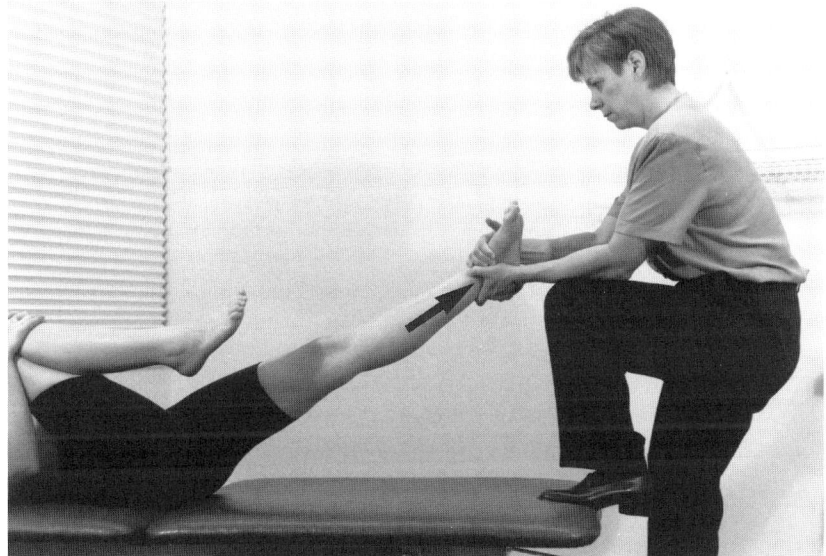

NOTES:

_____

_____

_____

_____

_____

_____

MANIPULATION TECHNIQUES — SACRUM

Subluxation of the sacrum – right anterior

Patient: Right sidelying, lower leg extended, upper hip and knee flexed.

Therapist: Standing facing the patient.

Localization: The thoracolumbar spine is rotated until L5-S1 is felt to be fully rotated to the left. The lateral aspect of the spinous process of the L5 vertebra is firmly stabilised with one thumb to maintain the rotation at the lumbosacral junction. With the index finger of this hand, palpate the right sacral base. With the other hand, rotate the left innominate bone and the locked lumbosacral unit to the right about a pure vertical axis through the pelvic girdle to the motion barrier of the right sacroiliac joint allowing the table to stabilise the right innominate bone.

Manipulation: From this position, a high velocity, low amplitude thrust is applied (arrow) through the left innominate bone and the sacrum to produce posterior translation of the right sacral base relative to the right innominate bone. The technique is followed by a re-evaluation of osteokinematic, arthrokinematic and arthrokinetic function.

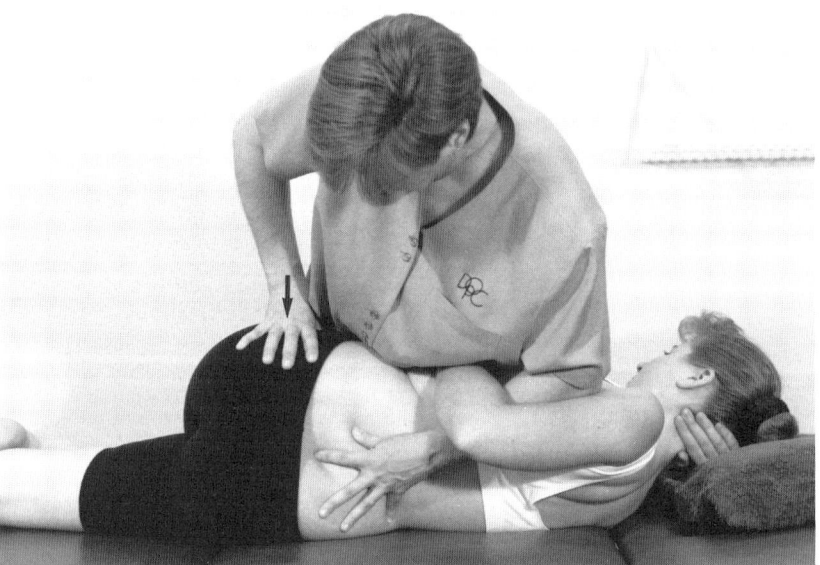

NOTES:

_____

_____

_____

MANIPULATION TECHNIQUES — SACRUM

Subluxation of the sacrum – right posterior

Patient:	Prone, with the right hip and knee flexed over the side of the table.
Therapist:	Standing on the patient's left side.
Palpate:	With the heel of the left hand, palpate the right sacral base. With the other hand, palpate the right iliac crest and the ASIS.
Manipulation:	Apply a posterior glide to the innominate against the fixed sacrum. When the motion barrier has been reached, a high velocity, low amplitude thrust is applied to the sacrum in an anterior direction. The technique is followed by a re-evaluation of osteokinematic, arthrokinematic and arthrokinetic function.

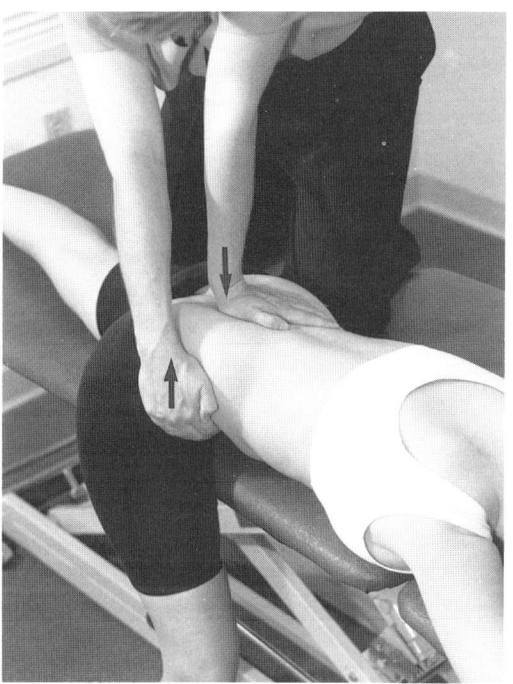

NOTES:

_____

_____

_____

_____

_____

_____

MANUAL THERAPY FOR THE THORAX

A biomechanical approach

DIANE LEE BSR MCPA COMP

Instructor/Chief Examiner for the Orthopaedic Division of the Canadian Physiotherapy Association

Acute and chronic thoracic pain is a common problem seen in physiotherapy practise today. There is very little anatomical, biomechanical or clinical research available for guidance in both evaluation and treatment planning. This text presents the osteoarticular anatomy and a biomechanical model of thoracic function. From this model, the objective examination for the painful thorax is developed.

The articular mobility and stability tests as well as the mobilization techniques are described and illustrated in detail. There are 191 illustrations. A stabilization program for instability is both illustrated and discussed. This text will become a very useful addition to the practising clinician's library.

Price: $40.00 (only prepayment can be accepted and we will cover all shipping and handling costs if posted to Canada. Out of country orders, please add $4.00 for shipping.)

To order, simply complete the form below and mail with your cheque/money order payable to DOPC to:

> DOPC – The Thorax
> 302 – 11950 80th Ave.,
> Delta, B.C.
> Canada, V4C 1Y2

.....cut here and return

Manual Therapy for the Thorax – a biomechanical approach by Diane Lee

Please send me _____ copies of this book.

Name: _____

Shipping address: _____